How to Save Your Life

EARL UBELL

How to Save Your Life

Harcourt Brace Jovanovich, Inc. / *New York*

Library of Congress Cataloging in Publication Data

Ubell, Earl.
  How to save your life.

  1. Hygiene. I. Title. [DNLM: 1. Hygiene—
Popular works. QT180 U13h 1973]
RA776.U23   613   73–7520
ISBN 0–15–142179–X

First edition
B C D E

To Shirley

I hope it all works

Contents

A Few Words That Go Before . . .

Usually I read prefaces and forewords after I finish reading a book, because only after I become entranced or disgusted with the writer do I wonder how he came to write at all. So, if you are like me, you already know why I wrote the book—the reason jumps out at you from chapter 1.

I should tell you I had an ego problem with this work. As a science reporter who made his reputation on being supercritical of scientists who purport to have discovered the cure for cancer, the cure for diabetes, the cure for schizophrenia, et cetera, I faced the dilemma of how to present the scientific evidence to support the suggestions on how to save your life. I could have footnoted nearly every statement with one or another of dozens of psychological, biological, and social observations. Such documentation would have made the book unreadable. On the other hand, by leaving out all references, the critic might seem uncritical. What to do!

I cast my lot with the reader. I am more interested in having the reader understand, accept, and apply what I have written than in proving everything I say with the rigor that belongs in a scientific journal. I can, however, back up what I say with scientific evidence, some weak, some strong, and I try to indicate how strong or how weak that evidence is. In places where I'm only guessing I say so. Faced with the problem of changing habits, however, a guess is better than nothing.

Inevitably, a book that takes two years to write will lag behind the ever-growing publication of scientific evidence. Some of my specific statements will fall under the weight of accumulating data; but most, I believe, will stand. In any case, if you follow the habit-forming recipes no harm can come to you: Is it bad to stop smoking? to change to a low-fat diet? to cut down on drinking? I don't think so, and neither do almost all physicians, psychologists, and public-health authorities.

I have taken the precaution of asking authorities in various fields to read certain chapters and to critique them for me. In that way I have eliminated the egregious errors, but if any remain they are my own recalcitrance or carelessness.

First, Dr. Cyril Franks, professor of psychology, Rutgers University, pointed the proper way in the behavioral aspects of this book (his was the most arduous task); Dr. Jeremiah Stamler, professor and chairman of community health and preventive medicine at Northwestern University, took on the diet and exercise chapters; Dr. Hans Kraus, professor of rehabilitation medicine at New York University, also went over the exercise chapter; Dr. Daniel Horn, of the National Clearing House of Tobacco and Health, read the smoking chapter; Dr. Dan Cahalan, professor of public health, and his colleagues, Dr. Robin Room and Dr. Ronald Roizen, of the Social Research Group at the School of Public Health of the University of California, dipped into the alcohol report; Dr. William Masters, of the Reproductive Biology Research Foundation, St. Louis, Dr. Joseph LoPiccolo, professor of psychology at the University of Oregon, and Ann Welbourne, of Community Sex Information, New York, all read the chapter on sex. To all of them, thanks.

Thanks, too, go to Ed Barber, for two years of friendly nagging and confidence; to Gloria Hammond, for an editing job I would have done myself if I had the guts; to Beverly Deaver, not only for typing the manuscript, but also for pointing out to me that in my maleness I may have overlooked aspects of femaleness in the sex chapter; to Gail Yancosek, for a hundred and one things that enabled me to finish the job; and to unnamed librarians at Cornell College of Medicine, Roosevelt Hospital, the College of Physicians and Surgeons, and the New York Public Library, for putting up with my impossible demands.

How to Save Your Life

1 / If You Want to Stay Alive

At first, you notice him only because he presses forward through the afternoon amblers with more speed than the rest. But as soon as he reaches an open space in the crowd, he breaks into a little jog, which rapidly slows to a jerky walk because he is quickly winded. Otherwise, he seems no different from many a small-businessman hurrying through the business district of any large city or small town in America. He is in a hurry to reach his bank before it closes, for he must make a deposit to cover a check he has drawn that day. As with many men who operate their own businesses, his days are filled with crises of insufficient funds. A shortage of $1,000 exerts the same psychic pressure on him as one of $1,000,000 does on a tycoon. He cannot countenance the faltering of his enterprise: he has a family—four sons, one just completing college, another high school, two others still small children. Besides, he believes he was made to succeed.

So he hurries along. Run . . . jog . . . walk . . . run . . . jog . . . walk. Now you notice that he is a short man, just about 5 feet 2 inches. And chubby . . . no, not chubby, really heavy. He will tell you that he weighs 155 pounds, but he actually carries 165 pounds. His forty extra pounds are more fat than muscle. Years ago, he played soccer; but he has not exerted himself physically in at least twenty years.

Now he stops for a moment. That lunch really bothers him: too greasy, he thinks. Corned beef sandwich, potato salad, coffee, and Danish pastry, all consumed quickly at his desk. While he has been eating such lunches forever with no ill effects, today it seems to be settling under his lungs as if congealed into stone. He glances up at the tower clock. He will make it now: five minutes before bank closing. On this hot June day, sweat pours down his back.

He lights a cigarette, pulls on it deeply, thinking that maybe it will dissolve the stone. Cigarettes often work that way for him. If he feels a little funny, he reaches for a cigarette and the peculiar feeling evaporates. That way he burns up three packs of Camels a day. This time the butt only makes him feel more peculiar; the stone seems heavier.

He starts to move again, but he cannot seem to lift his legs. That stone in his chest is growing. Then he feels that first huge stab of pain, as if a mason had brought his sledgehammer down to smash the stone. The blow strikes him to the ground and the windedness he felt before now gives way to gasping, as if he had been swimming and accidentally breathed in a cupful of water. Bang. Another blow of the sledgehammer.

The bank. He knows he must get there before it closes and he rises again (now there are hands helping him) but the stonemason is merciless. Even though he is sweating, he is cold and shivering. Then it dawns on him. He is having a heart attack. Its recurrence four days later would leave his forty-four-year-old heart a raw, hopeless, quivering mass of muscular rubble. In four days he would be dead.

Perhaps a million Americans meet the stonemason in this way each year; half do not survive the encounter. Not only businessmen, but men and women from all walks of life—rich, poor, professionals, laborers, whites, blacks, housewives, and career women. All have a style of life—eating, smoking, emotional pressure, lack of physical activity—that increases their chances of meeting the stonemason.

The scene replays itself in my mind often, because it is a real one to me. In 1948, it was played out by my father when he was forty-four years old and I was twenty-two. Having reached his age at this writing, I feel that the drama takes on a personal cogency. Moreover, having been a science reporter for twenty years and having studied the conditions of life and death, I feel an increasing obligation to my father's memory to help prevent the playing out of that scene for others. We are all in the grip of an epidemic. Unlike epidemics of the past, there is no bacterium, no virus. It is our very way of life that has ended millions of lives, not only those that, unlike my father's, had seemed to live themselves out, but those like his: young, bright, and brimming with future.

And heart attack is not the only villain. Cancer, drug addiction, alcoholism, accidents, sleeplessness, sex problems, and the aridity of growing old without much to do except sit on a park bench waiting for the stonemason—all must be added to the list. All arise, the scientific evidence suggests, from a way of life that is out of keeping with our biological inheritance. I am not talking about rare afflictions, like polio, muscular dystrophy, and multiple sclerosis, but rather those ailments that kill or incapacitate the majority of people they attack. And it seems we are doing these things to ourselves; trading the possibility of long, relatively disease-free lives for the pleasure of eating steak, smoking cigarettes, and blotting out cares with alcohol.

American affluence has conquered a host of infectious diseases by making it possible to live in relatively clean environments, with clean food and water. The high standard of living has confined the liabilities of outright hunger to a few pockets of poverty and, at the same time, provided magnificent comforts to which not even kings of old could aspire. Ironic, isn't it? An industrial revolution that extended our lives now cuts many short. Yours could be among them.

Consider: we ride, where our forebears ran or walked; we eat food gloriously rich in animal fats, while our ancestors subsisted on carbohydrates; we smoke cigarettes and provide our lungs with an intimate pollution of cancer-causing chemicals such as only chimney sweeps used to experience; our consumption of alcohol increases at such a rate as to make our supposedly hard-drinking pioneers seem like teetotalers; and we have gleefully taken up the products of the chemist's laboratory, consuming medicines and drugs by the ton and making the older consumption of morphine and opium in the heyday of Lydia Pinkham's Compound seem trivial by comparison. We seem intent on doing to ourselves what germs and viruses cannot.

We have the power to live longer and, more important, to live better. The two go hand in hand: long life and healthy life. But there are those—perhaps you are among them—who prefer to trade years for health. The inveterate cigarette smoker declares: "Okay: If I stop smoking I live four years longer. I like cigarettes enough to give up the four years."

He fails to realize that as a smoker the odds are he is going to be much sicker in the years before his early death than if he hadn't smoked at all. Life does not necessarily end with a thunderclap. Not everyone dies promptly, with a short spasm of pain, from a heart attack. More often, years of suffering will follow from chronic heart incapacity, for instance, or the drowning terrors of emphysema; if lung cancer intervenes, the victim's final illness will exhaust his and his family's financial resources. The American medical way is to pauperize individuals who have the misfortune to fall ill before they are sixty-five, when free medical care is finally available. By smoking, the average man has not traded four or eight years for the pleasure; he may have given up somewhere between ten and twelve years of living. What a price!

To me, and I hope to you, life is extraordinarily sweet, painful, exciting, boring, fulfilling, and frustrating—all at once. Yet I crave it as an addict craves his drug. I believe that the craving is general, that the most miserable person, the most downtrodden person, the most diseased person clutches upon every moment of life. Of those people who commit suicide—the ratio is less than one in a hundred—only a tiny fraction do so as a matter of rational decision. The rest are led to it by mental depressions over which they often have no conscious control.

A visitor from a distant universe would see millions of people, whose lives are threatened by illness, hanging on to every scrap of vitality. He would see a huge disease-treatment apparatus—doctors, nurses, hospitals, medicines—designed to provide sick people with extra weeks and months (rarely years) of life. He would recognize that individuals, having become ill and beset with pain and intimations of mortality, strive with every resource at their command to keep death away. Almost always the effort is too late.

At the same time, our unearthly visitor would see millions more of us, apparently healthy, scurrying heedlessly toward early disease and early death, doing things that, scientists now feel sure, shorten human life, make it less tolerable and ultimately more painful.

Individually and as a society, we have failed to recognize that the dramatic changes in our life styles have created new burdens on our health, and consequently we have failed to take any measures to preserve health and lengthen life. Many of us still hang on to the hope of a bygone, superstitious age, looking to physicians to provide magic potions or lay on the hands that will rescue us from our illnesses. We have operated on the principle that somebody will do something for us at the right time. Now, scientific research reveals that it is the person who is not yet ill, who is not yet a patient, who must do for himself.

Of course, it is not easy for us to think of ourselves as taking decisive action where our health is concerned—we are too used to relying on doctors and hospitals to rescue us from the results of carelessness about our health. But what about prevention of disease? Doctors do relieve pain, cure infections, and provide life-saving ministration. On the average, however, doctoring avails you little as far as life extension and life health are concerned, because prevention is not a primary characteristic of the doctor-patient relationship. A doctor's chief concern is cure, and cure rarely, if ever, controlled a disease. Prevention does.

It is interesting to examine briefly the history of one of the greatest advances made in the area of prevention, the increase of life expectancy. A male child born in 1900 had a 50-50 chance of living to age forty-eight. His life expectancy, which is an expression of probability only, not of certainty, was forty-eight years. A white male child born today, in 1973, has a life expectancy of nearly seventy years, an addition of nearly a quarter century. The gain among blacks has been even more dramatic: from thirty-three years for a black male born in 1900 to sixty-one years for one born today, a gain of twenty-eight years. Medical facilities available to blacks are enormously inferior to those available to whites, but there are other factors that keep black death rates high: poverty, crowding, poor diet, unsanitary conditions.

How was this increase in life expectancy accomplished? It is true that advances in scientific medicine and an increase in the number of hospitals paralleled the reduction of the death rate, but it would be incorrect to conclude that this was a matter of cause and effect. Let us look at this more closely. Up to the early part of the twentieth century, the major killers were infections; of these, tuberculosis took the biggest toll among young adults, diarrhea among infants. For nearly two centuries, public-health engineers and some physicians labored to improve the bacteriological quality of our environment: they cleaned up the water supply and eliminated cholera and typhoid fever. They pasteurized milk (a process invented by a French chemist), sanitized restaurants, collected garbage, installed sewer systems, established housing standards. At the same time, a rising affluence dramatically reduced crowding in homes, provided diets richer in protein and fresh vegetables, and improved working conditions.

The combined effect of these forces, none of them medical in the sense of treatment of patients, cut back death rates incredibly. In this country at the turn of the century, almost two out of every ten white and three out of ten black infants died before they reached their first year. Today fewer than three out of one hundred white babies and five out of one hundred black babies succumb—an almost tenfold improvement, and cleanliness, rather than doctoring, accounts for most of it.

In the beginning of this century, tuberculosis destroyed almost two hundred persons out of every one hundred thousand in the general population. Today, the TB death rate is about five per one hundred thousand. For that improvement, we should credit diet, general cleanliness, and reduction of crowding. There was no real treatment for tuberculosis until the discovery of streptomycin in 1947, when the death rate had already dropped 90 per cent.

Medicine gets major credit, however, for the development of vaccines to prevent diphtheria, whooping cough, and other infections. Such diseases—with the exception of polio—were already declining, thanks to the general cleanup; vaccines could now be counted as a strong addition to the list of preventive measures.

I have consistently challenged doctors to tell me of one treatment that eliminated a disease from a population. Usually, they cite penicillin for middle-ear infections, pneumonia, syphilis, and gonorrhea. One can accept the argument for middle-ear infections, which are now rare. But pneumonia, despite penicillin, still accounts for seventy thousand lives a year and the rate is quietly rising. Syphilis and gonorrhea, for which penicillin is almost an absolute cure, still persist; in fact, after a long decline, they are now increasing at an alarming rate. And while penicillin can make a strep throat disappear in a couple of days, the infection still cripples ten thousand children's hearts a year by inflaming the valves.

The sad fact is that now we only mouth the aphorism that an ounce of prevention is worth a pound of cure. Ever since we sanitized civilization and saved ourselves from infection, we pay only lip service to prevention.

The New Killers

With infections largely out of the way, a new set of ailments has achieved prominence: heart disease, cancer, emphysema, bronchitis, cirrhosis of the liver, and accidents. They account for nearly nine out of ten deaths and are the most painful and expensive events in our country. It is for these conditions that we have constructed that grand medical apparatus—doctors, nurses, hospitals, drugs, machines—in the vain attempt to control them. Yet these are the very diseases over which *you*, through preventive means, have potential control. It is you who must take the necessary steps in those aspects of your life style that foster development of those diseases. Only you can give yourself years.

There are many people who go to their doctors for an annual checkup in the hope of "picking up the signs of disease early." There is only meager evidence that annual physical checkups are a reductive factor in death or sickness rates. Even in the case of cancer, there is controversy, if not outright doubt, about the claim that early detection improves chances of surviving the disease. Reliance on annual physical checkups to keep your health is a slim reed on which to lean, though the reason is somewhat less than obvious. Those diseases against which the doctor and his medicines are powerful—infections—are promptly detectable by symptoms like fever and inflammation. Even if the doctor does not immediately use penicillins and mycins, they are powerful enough to make up for the delay in many cases. Streptococcal heart disease proves the point. In the wintertime children suffer from a variety of sore throats. Most are caused by various viruses; a small percentage by streptococci. If the physician promptly diagnoses the strep throat and uses penicillin, the infection clears up. If the infection, even though detected, is misdiagnosed as a virus infection, or for some other reason no treatment is applied, the strep spreads and in a significant number of cases does develop into rheumatic fever, with its potential crippling of the heart valves. Clearly, our social-medical structure is such that doctors miss a significant number of sore throats. The cure that is available is not applied. Unless every wintertime sore throat is carefully assessed, we shall continue to have crippled hearts.

On the other hand, the appearance of the signs of the big killers—heart, kidney, and other chronic ailments—is a signal that the disease has progressed substantially and will continue to do so in spite of what the physician does. For instance, if the arteries that carry blood to the heart muscle—the coronary arteries—are closed with fatty deposits, which brings on the painful symptoms of angina, the doctor may relieve the pain, but he can do almost nothing to clear those arteries, recent surgical techniques notwithstanding. Evidence of medical and physician impotence comes from the official disease tables: heart disease, cancer, cirrhosis of the liver, and accident death rates are all going up. A glance at the life-expectancy tables seems to reinforce that evidence.

Earlier, we spoke of the fantastic increases in life expectancy since 1900, when a baby had a 50-50 chance of living to forty-eight years. But let us ask the question, how long would a man be expected to live who was forty years old in 1900? Twenty-eight years, to age sixty-eight. Today, a forty-year-old man can expect, on the average, to live thirty-two more years, an improvement of only four years. What about the sixty-five-year-old man in 1900? His life expectancy was twelve years; today it is thirteen years. The point is, once a man gets safely through the infection period of childhood and youth and reaches middle age, he can expect to live to a tolerable old age. This was true in 1900 and it is true today. Medicine does little for those in middle and old age.

Extra Years, Extra Misery?

But who wants to live three years longer if they will be years of misery as a useless, senile vegetable? I have two reasons to believe that living longer can mean living better. One is that those dying young are sicker just before they die than those who die old. Think about it. Individuals die young today not because of a single event—a heart attack, a stroke, an overwhelming infection; they die after a period of considerable suffering from the new killers, which take a long time to develop. Before they die, old people are comparatively healthier; they spend less time in hospitals in the years preceding death. So it would appear that striving for long life by retarding the onset of disease also makes for a healthier, more productive life. This is especially true if the way in which one seeks that long life includes attention to diet, exercise, and achieving mental preparedness.

The great philosopher Pogo said that you never get out of this life alive. Death takes us all; none of us can buy or catch immortality. But *how* shall we die? Jonathan Swift, the seventeenth-century satirist, predicted that he would die like a tree, from the top down. Indeed, his brain was destroyed by what is now believed to have been syphilis. It seems to me that we, too, can, if not choose the exact manner of our death, at least decide whether we will die slowly over a number of years, failing in mind and body, or simply collapse at the end of a long, productive life, like the wonderful one-horse shay that came apart in a day.

Dr. Alex Comfort, a British physician and physiologist, has suggested that every mammalian species has an upper limit to its life span. It seems that horses, for instance, can live a maximum of fifty years, cats thirty, dogs twenty, rats five, elephants seventy, and human beings, the longest lived of all mammals, one hundred and ten years.

Of course, only a minute fraction of any species lives to the maximum. Human beings have only two chances in a thousand of living to be one hundred years old. Populations with the highest standards of living produce the most centenarians, because, with infection conquered, there are more survivors who have the biological capacity to reach the century mark. However, most people fall short of the maximum, victims either of inborn weaknesses that do not show up until later years or of their own failure to take proper advantage of their natural capacities. Up until recent years little was known about achieving long life. Now biological studies are providing an ever-increasing wealth of helpful information. Evidence collected by Dr. Comfort indicates that the closer an individual gets to the maximum life span, the less illness he experiences. And this is just one inspiring fact enabling us to hope that one day our bodies may indeed behave more like the one-horse shay. As we work toward extending our life expectancy, we will, I believe, simultaneously extend our physical and mental well-being, our productivity, and our enjoyment; then, when death does intervene, it will be quick and clean.

What We Have to Know

An increasing number of human-biology studies are showing a connection between disease and early death, on the one hand, and the way we live, on the other. Most Americans understand the connection; indeed, they probably feel not a little guilty about the way they eat, drink, and live. But in spite of the understanding and the guilt, they do not change their habits. Is it because they do not care about what they are doing to themselves? I do not think so. Anybody who is confronted with the real possibility of disease or death cares passionately. Witness the vast expenditure of money—$70 billion in 1971 and growing at 10 per cent a year—to thwart death, to heal affliction. Nothing is more pathetic than the family of a man with lung cancer emptying out their bank accounts, mortgaging their future, in the vain attempt to buy him a few more weeks of life. They want to feel they have done everything at the end. So people do care. Why, then, don't they change their life styles?

Part of the answer lies in the fact that people untroubled by ill health are convinced of the invincibility of their present state of well-being. One ice-cream cone or a steak could hardly be a threat. Then, too, any unfortunate results of their life style seem to lie in a far-distant future; it is difficult to believe in negative possibilities. But I think the largest part of the answer lies in the fact that our life styles are an orchestration of many habits. Recent experiments in behavioral psychology have led to the discovery that our life styles are deeply imbedded habits, as deeply imbedded as an addiction to drugs. The process that leads to drug addiction, which modern theory sees as mainly psychological rather than biological, bears strong resemblance to the process that leads to overeating, becoming sedentary, and performing the thousand and one daily acts that constitute a life style.

In order to increase the chances of living a longer and better life, scientists are now combining the discoveries of biology with those of psychology. Biology studies tell us what areas of our lives must change if we want to preserve health; behavioral-psychology studies provide a range of techniques that you can apply toward changing your life style: to stop or reduce smoking, to start—and to continue—exercising, to lose weight, to change the kind of food you eat, to avoid the traps of accidents, to prevent overuse of mood-changing medicine, to decrease alcohol consumption, to find sleep, to improve your sexual life, and to prepare for an old age that will be filled with interest and vitality rather than a constant fear of death.

There is no guarantee that if you follow the recipes in this book you will live longer or better. You will, however, increase your chances of doing so. To this reasoning some people would reply: "Okay. Just suppose I stopped smoking to live longer. I could walk across the street tomorrow and get killed by an automobile. So, no thank you, I'll keep on smoking and enjoy myself."

Such an assertion might have had more relevance in past centuries, when death rates from infection, war, and accident ran high, when it was indeed only a matter of fortune, good or ill, that determined survival. But, as we have already seen, this is the century in which individuals may be able greatly to influence their biological futures and seek the maximum life span.

I would love to play dice with the kind of fellow who believes totally in fate and luck and does not understand probability and odds or, if he does, chooses to ignore them. Against such a player, I win all the money. And if he plays that way in life, he loses, too. To believe that the odds of being killed crossing the street are equal to those of being killed through smoking is making the dice player's mistake of betting against the odds.

About ten thousand pedestrians meet death yearly. About fifty thousand persons die of lung cancer each year. If only half the lung cancers were caused by cigarettes (it is likely more), the chances would be $2\frac{1}{2}$ to 1 that you would kill yourself with lung cancer caused by smoking cigarettes before you would be killed crossing the street.

Doing for Yourself

This book is dedicated to showing you how to do for yourself—how to lengthen your life and improve its mental and physical quality. If every man and woman applied the knowledge now available, they could improve life expectancy by about eight or ten years on the average, while greatly reducing the burdens of disease, pain, and misery.

This is a book for normal people of normal intelligence who are healthy; it is not for those who are already sick. They should go to doctors, for they will not find any way to cure disease here. It is a book for those who appear healthy but are actually on a collision course with premature disease and death and do not know it or even suspect it. Who are they? Let me give you some facts about the person who is steering toward that collision. He or she:

• Carries at least 15 per cent extra weight.

• Eats beef, lamb, or pork at least once a day; consumes tabs of butter; puts cream in coffee; drinks whole milk; revels in gobs of ice cream; and eats hard cheese.

• Rarely gets any exercise except pushing a pencil, lifting a fork, or working a vacuum cleaner.

• Smokes at least a pack of cigarettes a day.

• Drinks four or more ounces of hard liquor, a pint of wine, or a couple of quarts of beer a day.

• Pops pep pills, sleeping pills, or tranquilizers in perceptibly *increasing* amounts.

• Handles his automobile on the road as if it were a kiddy car in a playground.

If all of these statements fit you, it is quite probable that your life will be short and not as happy as it could be. Your chances of surviving to the age of fifty are just about 50-50.

Fortunately, the average American can boast only one or two of these life-destroying proclivities. But even with one, his risk of early death goes up. Depending on which habit you have and to what degree you have it, your potential loss of life can range up to ten years. Multiple bad habits simply increase the risk. More important, the loss of living years, years without disease, may be even greater.

It is true that many individuals treat themselves as if their health were invulnerable and still live long and relatively unafflicted lives. Their favorite rejoinder to a cautionary remark is some variation of: "I had a great-uncle who smoked and drank and ate until he was ninety." You do inherit a tendency to longevity. Your chances of achieving old age are high if your grandparents lived to advanced years. But don't count on it; you won't know if you have inherited their good fortune until you get there. Remember that there are no certainties, only probabilities. If your life style includes any of the "bad" habits, you are decreasing your odds of living longer and better, even if you have "good" heredity.

There is a catch to doing for yourself. It involves changing lifelong habits of pleasure: smoking, drinking, hearty eating, to name the three most prominent. Few vigorous, healthy young people want to undertake the arduous changing of their present, enjoyable life style for some future, perhaps unattainable, benefit.

Besides, in the present climate of searching for bizarre experiences, of doing one's thing, of living for the moment, it may sound square to be reaching for health and long life. Ironically, those who ignore responsibility for their health by playing reckless roulette with their biological endowment later think nothing of burdening society or family with the results of that irresponsibility by asking them to pay for their medical care. Today, medical care is a shared responsibility; nobody pays for his own lung cancer or heart attack without a major contribution from the rest of us.

Enjoy, Enjoy

Is it really possible for you to change your life style—something you now enjoy, or at least say you enjoy—for some future benefit? Especially when you are happier eating thick steaks, puffing cigarettes, or even turning on with marijuana, than you would be by eliminating these enjoyables and adding some years to your life? I think it is, once you understand that most things in life you enjoy you have learned to enjoy. Indeed, it is possible to teach yourself to replace your current sources of pleasure with new ones. Perhaps the most important result of this process will be your discovery that your former enjoyables no longer appeal to you.

2 / The Theory and Practice
of Life Style

I used to be a big steak-and-potatoes man, capable of wolfing down a twelve-ounce steak at a sitting and enjoying every mouthful. Of course I was 30 per cent overweight, and God knows the condition of my arteries. Then I drastically reduced my consumption of animal fat and switched to fish and fowl. Not only did I begin to enjoy fish and fowl, but when I would occasionally try a twelve-ounce steak, I no longer enjoyed it, nor could I finish it.

Think about cigarette-smoking. When a youngster starts smoking, he coughs, gags, and feels woozy, hardly an enjoyable experience. Then, step by step, he teaches himself to discern the effect of nicotine beyond the irritation and to enjoy the lift the drug gives him. Were it not for the social pressures that influence young people to smoke, I do not think they would take it up; certainly they would not continue it voluntarily.

I can assure you that if you change your life style by changing your habits, as suggested in this book, your new set of habits will be as enjoyable as your old set. The transition will be rough. It will require hard psychic and physical work to change; there are no pills, no potions, few short cuts.

By their very nature habits are things we do not think about. But a moment's reflection will convince you that habits—good ones—are the liberators of your daily life, opening the way to intellectual and emotional freedom. The day-to-day dressing, eating, talking, and working would enervate the most durable person if he had to think through each action and make conscious choices at each step. Imagine what tying your shoelaces would be like if you had to figure out the method of tying the knot each time. Automatic behavior—habit—frees the creative parts of the brain.

How often have we seen individuals whom we call "highly organized" breeze through a job that we know would take us hours of torture to accomplish? Such people have simply arranged their lives into well-patterned habits, which usually include set times for carrying out intellectual projects, often in early morning. Geniuses almost always have highly patterned work habits; high productivity is usually one hallmark of genius.

Skinner Boxes and Pigeons

To find out how to form and to change habits, we will examine some of the findings of behavioral psychology, especially in reference to learning theory. Dr. B. F. Skinner, of Harvard University, is the father of modern behavioral psychology. His work has led to developments in programmed learning, theories of obesity and drug and alcohol addiction.

In programmed learning, a student is given some information and then asked a question about that information. If he answers incorrectly, he is given the correct answer immediately; if he answers correctly, he goes on to the next portion of information. Studies of the method indicate that it conveys information at least as well as a teacher can but at far less cost. Using a "Skinner Box" and a pigeon, I demonstrated to my own satisfaction an example of programmed learning, that is, the establishment of an automatic and persistent pattern of behavior.

Inside the Skinner Box was a pigeon and a feeding station with a trap door over it. The pigeon was hungry. As the bird pouted and strutted about the cage, I watched for it to approach the door. When it did, I hit a switch that opened the feeder. The pigeon pecked at the corn a couple of times. Then I closed the feeder. The pigeon loitered near the door, "encouraged" by the feeding. I have used quotes here to indicate a word that a behaviorist would not use to describe what was happening. He would say that the provision of the reward (the food) following a behavior (loitering near the door) increases the probability of the behavior's recurring. It is not necessary to go into psychological reasons. The pigeon is regarded simply as an organism that behaves in a particular way. (Recently, however, there has been a good deal of work on brain function in order to get at the physiological phenomena that accompany the reward-behavior mechanism.)

I waited until the pigeon turned his body a couple of degrees to the right (a random movement during his strutting) before opening the feeding station for him again. And after each subsequent feeding I waited until he turned more and more to the right before opening the trap door. I never rewarded left turning. Within ten minutes I had him making a complete circle to the right after each feeding. He continued for an hour after I stopped feeding him. He had formed a habit. Thus, repeated reward for behavior not only increases the probability of the recurrence of the behavior; it may make the behavior automatic in response to a signal.

Psychologists now believe that in the formation of a habit, the power of reward is great among all animal species. Among human beings, the rewards come from society, which approves desired behavior with affection, congratulations, grades, money, et cetera. Unlike most animals, human beings respond to symbolic rewards, to ideas and to certain emotions, and thus can form habits of behavior at much higher levels. Speech is an automatic behavior that is formed by a reward system, although reward does not entirely account for the phenomenon. Humans are biologically wired for speech, but the reward system shapes the speech pattern. It is also becoming increasingly clear that the habitual use of alcohol, drugs, excess food, as well as habits of sexual activity, often arises from a reward/behavior mechanism as formed within a particular social context.

Systematic use of reward to shape behavior has resulted in the formation of desirable (and often undesirable) habits in schoolchildren, and in controlling dieting and cigarette-smoking. It has also been used successfully in schools for the retarded. There, scientists have set up dispensers that deliver a piece of candy to a patient when he engages in desired behavior. If he works steadily at a task, he receives his reward at specified intervals; if he turns from the task, to fight with a nearby patient, for instance, no candy comes forth. The result has been quieter workrooms, less fighting, and indications that the patients are happier. In many institutions severe punishments are used to obtain the same behavior as can now be obtained with a few pieces of candy.

Punishment, of course, can be an important ingredient in getting rid of a habit, as we all know from our childhoods. In human beings, however, punishment can have unwanted side effects unless it is carefully used. Psychologists have tried applying electric shock to break habitual alcohol intake. But, while alcohol intake is reduced, the patient often becomes extremely hostile to the doctor and to those around him. Punishment usually works faster but, in the long run, reward works better.

Have you ever noticed how many stimuli, or signals, there are in daily life? Much of our automatic behavior occurs in response to external and internal signals. We get up in the morning when the alarm clock rings. We swallow food when we have chewed it to a certain consistency. We step on the accelerator of the car when the light changes from red to green. Often unconsciously, we perform daily a whole repertoire of automatic responses, or habits. When you begin to use the laws of habit your job will be to institute the proper automatic behavior after certain signals and also to quash certain of your existing responses.

I have so far steered away from technical terms to explain behavior modification and I will try to continue that practice. For example, instead of "reward" psychologists often use "positive reinforcement." But the word reward is not only good enough for explanation; it is also an instant reminder of what one must do. You may also have heard phrases like "operant conditioning," "desensitization," "reciprocal inhibition," and "stimulus-response." As useful as they are to the scientist, they may confuse the beginner and so retard his use of the practical results of psychological research.

The example of pigeon-training has illustrated the general idea of habit formation. You are now ready to examine the laws of habit-learning. All of them are based on psychological-research data. You will see how these laws can be used as the basis of any life-style-change program that you adopt in order to better your health.

The Laws of Habit, Using Reward

1 / If a reward *immediately follows* a particular behavior, that behavior will most likely recur. The pigeon in the box and the retarded children are illustrations of this. It is one of the strongest laws, established as unquestionably true for humans and for almost all other animal species.

You can use this law on yourself by paying yourself off in a pleasant way for work that is unpleasant. Thus if you find lawn-mowing not to your liking, you should always follow it with something pleasant.

Corollary: If you reward a behavior in the presence of a signal, the behavior will recur in response to the signal without the reward. Thus by sounding a bell as I simultaneously fed the pigeon, I could have made him pirouette simply by giving the signal—the bell. Actually the sequence has to be: bell—turn—feed, or, in psychological terms: signal—behavior—reward.

You can use this on yourself. Suppose you have trouble getting up in the morning. You set the alarm, but then you reach over and shut it off and go back to sleep. Instead, you should have the alarm across the room with something pleasant near it: orange juice, hot tea, coffee, cocoa in a Thermos jug—or anything you really like. Then, *after* you have gotten up but *before* you shut the alarm off, take a sip of the drink. After a few mornings, you should find getting up easier.

2 / It is possible to increase the frequency of infrequent behavior by following it with high-frequency behavior. A low-frequency behavior is some act that rarely happens by itself that you want to make automatic; a high-frequency behavior is something you do often and may already be a habit by itself.

So far, the word reward has been used to describe something obviously pleasant. But the reward need not be pleasant in the obvious way. For example, if you watch a mouse in a cage that has a vertical merry-go-round, you will notice that the animal runs on the merry-go-round frequently. You cannot say that the mouse "likes" to run; such concepts are beyond scientific provability. You can only say that the mouse does a lot of running on that merry-go-round. Suppose you now allow the mouse to use the merry-go-round only *after* he takes a sip of water. You can arrange it so that as he sips the water, a door in a wall separating him from the merry-go-round opens. The surprising thing is that the mouse now drinks much more water. The merry-go-round running has reinforced—"rewarded"—water-drinking.

In a sense, the second law is more powerful, or at least more useful, than the first because it does not necessitate thinking in terms of reward. All you need to do is observe your daily activities and find one that occurs frequently enough to be used as a reward. This law also raises the possibility of pyramiding habits, that is, using one habit to form a second and using the second to form a third.

The law has been demonstrated in the following experiment. Children are led one by one into a room that contains a dispenser of small chocolate candies and a pinball machine. They can play with either one. The children fall naturally into two groups: players and eaters. When it was arranged that a player could use the pinball machine only if he took a candy first, his eating increased; his playing, however, did not decline. With eaters, the playing went up when they were told they must play before eating; the eating was not less frequent. For one group, the frequent behavior of playing acted as a reward; for the other group it was eating.

The second law is of great practical importance, particularly in the control of eating—one doesn't want to use food as a reward for not eating! I have used the law myself, consciously and with modest success. Not long ago, I had a very sloppy desk at my office, despite a great desire to keep it orderly; occasional great bursts of cleaning zeal never made much of a difference. So I examined my daily activities to see what sort of high-frequency activity I engaged in. It took about three seconds to think of the telephone, which at that time I used about forty times a day. I decided to become my own pigeon. I would perform at least one desk-cleaning act before using the telephone or even answering it. My desk became neater than before. I will even let the telephone ring while I shift a piece of paper. More than that, I can see that the behavior is automatic. Often I am lost in thought and the telephone rings. I find myself reaching for a piece of paper rather than the telephone.

Corollary: A human being can arrange the contingencies, the rewards, the activities of his life in order to get desired behavior from himself. No other animal can do this. Along with speech and symbolic thinking, this ability is a hallmark of our human character. We simply have not used it consciously enough in the past, often allowing ourselves to become habituated to an activity merely by chance. Now, using the techniques of behavioral psychology, we can choose the habits we need.

3 / The power of programmed learning lies in the reward or high-frequency behavior following *immediately* upon the task. Although this law is imbedded in the first and second laws, I have stated it separately in order to emphasize its importance. Reward will not work at all if it arrives long after the desired behavior. That is why school grades that come at the end of the term are weak behavior reinforcements, as are test grades returned at the end of a week or even a day.

All the research on programmed learning indicates that it helps the student to learn information by himself at about the same rate he would if he had a teacher. Of course, teachers do not only provide information; they present a certain style and attitude toward it that can be just as important as the information itself. In times of teacher shortages, it might be helpful to use programmed learning for the acquisition of information, while leaving to teachers what they can do best: providing a style and attitude.

4 / Once the pattern of desired behavior is established, the frequency of the reward should be randomly reduced. Animals that have been trained on random-reward systems keep their habits much longer than do animals that have been rewarded every time for a desired behavior.

In other words, if I had tossed a coin, rewarding my pigeon on heads and not rewarding him on tails when he performed the turn, the bird would have turned without reward for many hours. I am not talking of rewarding the bird every other time. If you toss a coin you get a random sequence of heads and tails like this: heads, tails, heads, tails, tails, tails, heads, tails, et cetera. The average would turn out to be 50 per cent heads, 50 per cent tails, but no given toss could be predicted either way.

Gambling is an illustration of the firmness of habits created by random reward. A gambler sometimes wins and sometimes loses. The pay-off is completely random. The random-reward mechanism is a powerful force in turning a habitual gambler into an addict. It is also what keeps a research scientist in his laboratory around the clock. He never knows when there is going to be a pay-off. More than one scientist hooked on his work has actually reported psychic discomfort when he was not in his laboratory. Random reward. It's very powerful.

No damage is done if occasionally we reward ourselves when we have not performed the desired behavior. This is especially cogent for dieters: breaking a diet may prove more effective in the long run than trying to stick to one eating pattern. Tossing a coin to see if one should reward oneself could be a powerful technique to instill a habit. It's worth trying.

5 / The low-frequency nonautomatic behavior must precede the high-frequency automatic act. In other words, you cannot put the reward *before* the desired behavior.

If you want to form the habit of putting on your automobile seat belt, you should put on the seat belt before you turn the ignition key or, even better, before you put the key into the ignition lock. In getting into the habit of keeping my desk neat, it would have done no good at all if I had cleaned it after telephoning. (For salesmen who are loath to make telephone calls but good at shuffling papers, the technique would be to telephone before shuffling.)

6 / A human being is capable of rewarding himself *mentally* for performing a desired behavior. This is particularly practical for inducing habits for which there may be no handy overt behavior that can be used for a reward.

It works something like this: you think of a pleasant scene— swimming on a hot day, ocean waves rolling in, sipping a good cup of coffee, walking hand in hand with somebody you love, chatting with a friend—any scene at all, as long as it is pleasant to you. Then you conjure up the scene after you have performed the behavior you want to habitualize. If I wanted to use it for the sloppy-desk problem, I should first perform a desk-cleaning act and then pause and think of that pleasant scene.

For this method to be effective, you must make the pleasant thought a high-frequency act, and this may be difficult at first. Psychologists have worked out a do-it-yourself technique for practice: lie on a couch as relaxed as possible and say to yourself a key word that will make you think of the pleasant scene. Repeat this many times until you have no trouble imagining the scene. Dwell on it . . . it is pleasant. The sequence should be:

You say to yourself: Reward.

You think: Walking arm in arm with someone you like along a beautiful beach.

Your thoughts wander.

You repeat: Reward.

The scene returns.

After a few days of practice you will be able to make the scene appear instantly, and you will then have a useful tool with which to form any habit. It is particularly useful in learning to enjoy new foods that are better for your body than the foods you now eat, and in acquiring the exercise habit.

Corollary: When people think well of what they have done, they usually do the same things again. Some psychologists believe that self-congratulation can be used formally as a reward. If you perform the behavior you want to make a habit, you say to yourself, Terrific. Atta boy (or girl, as the case may be)—or any phrase that tells you that you have done well.

I know that some people may be self-conscious in using such ideas. It seems a little mechanistic, as do, indeed, all the ideas of habit formation. Yet there is good evidence to show that persons who are self-approving in schoolwork do better in school than those who are not. Moreover, students in the presence of teachers who are self-approving model themselves after their teachers. So if such processes happen naturally and are effective, why not use them to form a life style?

Generally, reward is a more desirable technique for habit control. In breaking habits, however, it is often possible to make efficient use of self-punishment. Since results come rapidly the general motivation to change the life style can be sustained. For instance, a person's signal to eat might be a recurring situation that makes him nervous. Building a new habit that inhibits eating may take a few months by using reward, and the possibility of a bad situation occurring in that interval is high. On the other hand, if in a few weeks one can instill a new regime by using punishment, it may be possible to make the new habit strong before the adverse situation intervenes.

The Laws of Habit, Using Punishment

1 / Punishment is effective in extinguishing behavior if it follows immediately after or is coincident with the undesired behavior.

Anybody who has trained a puppy not to urinate in the house knows that the main difficulty is to catch the dog just as he performs the act. If one waits too long to punish him, he winds up confused. For people, punishment is often simply being reminded that they are engaging or are about to engage in unwanted acts.

A number of my secretaries were once nail biters. When I asked if they wished to stop, they all said yes, but they couldn't seem to.

I instructed each to buy some bitter-tasting product like Thum or Bitex, available at the drugstore, and paint it on their nails. I then told them that every time one of them painted her nails with the anti-nail-biting material, I would pay her a penny. I thereby rewarded the preferred behavior—nail-painting. Many parents who want to make their children stop biting nails or sucking thumbs make the mistake of painting the child's nails or fingers. It is much better to get the child to do the painting by rewarding him for it and explaining what you are doing. That way you give him a technique for behavior control. The punishment comes not only from the bitter taste, but from the knowledge that he is engaging in undesirable behavior that is in conflict with the desired behavior (painting the nails).

I have tried the method with four of my secretaries and failed only once, with a woman who was in psychotherapy. She felt uncomfortable with what she called a "mechanistic" approach to behavior. She had to know why she was biting her nails before she would stop. She hasn't found out why yet, or if she has, it has not helped her to stop biting. The other women still don't know why they bit their nails, but they now have beautifully manicured hands.

Corollary: Punishment is especially effective if it comes immediately after the signal that starts the unwanted behavior and just before the behavior actually starts.

This is important, because it is necessary to develop the strength to withstand signals, rather than get away from them. If the sight of ice cream stimulates the eating behavior of a person who must change his diet, the chances are high in our society that he will frequently encounter ice-cream signals. It is at just those times that punishment is more efficient than reward, because it is often easier to establish a punishment strong enough to thwart the onset of eating than it is to provide a reward for not eating while the signal is present.

The same principle applies to the drug problem. It is easy enough to keep an addict drug free in an institution where there are no drugs. But once he returns to the drug-using environment, the signals for use abound: friends who use drugs, the actual sight of drugs, and anxieties arising from trying to cope with life situations. Most drug-treatment programs suffer from the fact that they do not provide either reward or punishment in the presence of a drug-use signal. And indeed, drugs themselves provide such powerful rewards that it is difficult to arrange other rewards or punishments that will be powerful enough to counter the drug response. Because the nicotine in cigarettes acts like a drug in some people, it is particularly difficult for them to stop smoking, even though they have a strong desire to.

2 / As with reward, it is better not to punish every undesired act.

I did not make a big fuss when the women forgot to paint their nails and nibbled at their fingers a little. As long as the majority of the unwanted acts are punished, the technique works. In fact, a few misses improve things.

3 / Punishment before the behavior fails if it precedes the signal that sets the behavior in motion.

Prespanking children for expected misbehavior simply doesn't work and produces hostility.

Corollary: Punishment long after the undesired behavior is relatively ineffective; the longer you wait, the less the effect.

4 / A human being is capable of punishing himself mentally.

Like the comparable law on pleasant thoughts, this concept is of great practical importance. It provides a handy, always available method of self-punishment. There are reports that the use of unpleasant thoughts as punishment can reduce homosexual behavior, heavy drinking, and cigarette-smoking. In my personal experience it worked to terminate habits I wanted to end. As with pleasant thoughts, it requires practice.

What are some examples of unpleasant thoughts? Perhaps a vision of yourself as too fat to go through a door (as a control for eating), a picture of your lungs turned blood black (as a control for smoking), or of yourself as a gray corpse (for drinking). The unpleasant thought need not be true; it need only be an image that is connected in your mind with the bad habit you wish to end.

Suppose, for instance, you do not wish to eat bread at the dinner table—it is right there, signaling you to eat. As you feel yourself reaching for the bread, but before you actually do, flash into your mind that picture of yourself as too fat to move through a door. It should momentarily stop the feeling of wanting the bread. Immediately take a sip of water and engage somebody in conversation. It does work. You'll find yourself eating less and less bread.

Automatic Behavior

A habit is automatic behavior that has been set in motion by some sort of signal. Signals are important in helping us to understand our life styles. They can be external: the traffic light changes to green, we step on the accelerator. We do not think about it; we just do it in response to the signal. In such activities we bear a striking resemblance to the pigeon in the Skinner Box.

Some signals are internal, hunger pangs for instance. Much scientific research has been done in an effort to elaborate the origin of hunger signals. They appear to arise through a complex interaction involving an empty stomach, changing sugar levels in the blood, some sort of internal timekeeping mechanism, and certain sections of the brain. There are satiety signals of a similar nature. Recent evidence suggests that overweight individuals pay less attention to these than do persons of normal weight.

Some signals are complex. You are in a conversation with your boss. He is being mildly critical of something you have done. It makes you nervous (the posher word is "anxious"), and you reach automatically for your cigarettes. You have set off a train of behavior that is unstoppable until you draw that first puff. That feeling of nervousness was the signal for initiating the smoking behavior. The anxiety is internal, but it is initiated by an external situation.

The psychologist calls a signal a "stimulus." In our lives, we respond to all sorts of internal and external stimuli that govern such automatic behavior as eating, drinking, smoking, sleeping, and sexual activity. The stimuli include sights (food), sounds (sleep), odors (food and sex), touch, temperature, clocks, light levels, specific words. Very few give us a choice of behavior. Once the specific stimulus to which we have learned to respond appears, the chances are very high that we will begin a specific repertoire of behavior. It takes practice to recognize the presence of a given stimulus. With certain habits—like eating, smoking, alcohol-drinking, drug-taking, sleeping—the stimulus-response dyad is so strong that most people find it impossible not to respond without some very special effort to intervene after the stimulus and before the behavior occurs.

How does one modify the strong stimulus-response chains? The laws of reward/punishment provide, I believe, the best chance of making modifications. They will not always succeed, because they require conscious preparation and consistent application. And for many people with life-style habits that are harmful, emotional reasons prevent the application of these methods. For example, in certain individuals the mood-modifying qualities of alcohol are rewarding enough to nullify any other possible self-reward or self-punishment that he may propose. Similar effects may occur with eating, smoking, drug-taking, and sleeping. For such people, a modest amount of outside help from a parent, friend, spouse, or even an employer may turn the trick by providing the rewards and punishments in a sufficiently consistent manner to overcome the rewarding nature of the bad habit. You will find in this book specific suggestions on how to get that outside help, but of course, if you can do it yourself, you will have developed a powerful psychological tool for use as you see fit.

When a particular habit has become so strong that the person's entire way of life has become involved with it, that person has an addiction. Any attempt to change the addiction carries a high risk of relapse. I suspect that anybody who is 50 per cent or more overweight is a food addict. Individuals who smoke more than two packs a day are probably nicotine addicts. Similarly, there is a good chance that those who drink four to six ounces of alcohol a day (that is, five to eight ounces of liquor, five to eight four-ounce glasses of wine, or five to eight cans of beer) are either already addicted (alcoholic) or on their way. Finally there are those who find that every day they must take amphetamines (pep pills) to get started, tranquilizers to calm down, or barbiturates to get to sleep. They are probably addicted.

While it is not scientifically rigorous to define addiction in terms of quantity of food, cigarettes, alcohol, or drugs, quantity is a useful guide in determining addiction. An older definition—widely held both by the medical profession and by laymen—holds that addiction is present only when the withdrawal of the drug produces physical symptoms. Yet one can become addicted to amphetamines or cocaine without physical withdrawal symptoms. A better definition holds that an addict is a person whose major preoccupation is with obtaining and using the particular substance, and who, deprived of the substance, searches relentlessly for it. This book cannot really help such addicts, although I do believe that the principles of reward and punishment can be applied by physicians and psychologists in their treatment of addiction. Few of them do; the former tend to rely on medical treatment, while the latter favor psychological methods that are geared more to understanding the origin of addiction than to reshaping behavior.

The essential features of desirable or undesirable habit formation are:

1. A signal is perceived by you (word command, the sight of a cookie, an argument with your wife).

2. You perform a behavior immediately after the signal (you tie a shoelace, eat a cookie, smoke a cigarette).

3. A reward follows the act almost immediately (praise, diminished hunger, less anxiety).

4. This sequence occurs many times, although No. 3 (reward) need not follow No. 2 (performance) every time.

5. You can use the above four steps in forming a new habit. Remember, a thought can be used as a reward.

To break a habit, the following steps are necessary:

1. Identify the stimulus that starts your train of behavior (food on the table, nervousness at work, the cocktail hour).

2. Avoid the stimulus until it no longer produces the response or—better but more difficult—

3. In the presence of the stimulus, inhibit the train of behavior that it sets off (food is present but you do not eat; you feel nervous but do not smoke; at a cocktail party you do not drink).

4. You can help yourself achieve step 3 by a combination of punishment and reward—punishment to inhibit the behavior you want to stop, reward for having achieved the inhibition. Again, remember that thoughts, good and bad, can be used as rewards and punishments.

5. Repeat steps 3 and 4 until the habit has disappeared.

Notice that neither habit formation nor habit-breaking requires you to know the reason for the behavior—such reasons as "I smoke because I'm self-destructive"; "I eat because I'm sexually frustrated"; "I don't like fish because my mother used to force it on me." They are part of a psychological method different from the one presented in this book. Complex ideas like Oedipal relations and abreactions can be valid in explaining the origin of the habit, but they may not explain its continuation or be of use in discontinuing it.

For example, a child wets his bed because his mother made him angry and upset by spanking him for breaking a dish. His emotional disturbance causes him to lose control of his urinary sphincter, the muscle that opens and closes the tube leading from the bladder. In the morning, his mother becomes angry with him again, this time for wetting his bed. When he goes to sleep that night she threatens punishment if he wets. Again anger and frustration weaken his control, and again in the morning his mother is angry.

The child now realizes he has control over his mother. He can make her angry. Her anger becomes a reward for his wetting. The punishment she inflicts comes too long *after* the actual event—the bed-wetting—to be an effective inhibitor of the act. So each night at an internal signal—a full bladder—his sphincter relaxes. The reward he gets *after* the act, control of his mother, is effective in habitualizing the behavior.

Perhaps after a year or two, the mother seeks psychological counseling and as a result calms down. The disturbed relations between parent and child subside, but the bed-wetting persists. Why? One can give complex psychological reasons, but the reward/punishment theory suffices. Bed-wetting has been habitualized. It occurs automatically with the appearance of the stimulus: pressure in the bladder. Since it occurs while the child is asleep, he can make no conscious effort of will to control it.

To stop bed-wetting, it is only necessary to wake the child just as the act begins. He needs a reminder—a mild punishment—to inhibit the train of events. It is quite similar to the situation in nail-biting. In this case, a wire mesh is placed under the sheet. As soon as the first drops of fluid touch the wire, a switch is closed and a bell or buzzer rings, waking the child and permitting him to consciously control the situation. After a few nights and a few awakenings, the new habit takes over: control of the sphincter. Soon he no longer wets and he no longer awakens. The method has been tested and is highly successful, more so than any approach that emphasizes "understanding" the reasons for the wetting.

The Case for Learning Theory

All the laws of habit formation and change are based on findings of the branch of psychology known as learning theory. Developed from the results of experiments with animals and human beings, the theory is reflected in the work of Ivan Pavlov, a Russian physiologist, and of the American psychologists John Watson and B. F. Skinner.

In the early years of the twentieth century, Pavlov clearly demonstrated that a behavior (in this case, salivation) brought on in the presence of one stimulus (food) could be brought on by another stimulus (a bell) if the second were made to appear in conjunction with the first. Thus Pavlov was able to cause a dog to salivate merely at the sound of the bell. In 1920, Watson showed he could instill fear in a child with a white rat, which normally did not alarm him, by showing the rat to the child while at the same time doing something that did frighten the child. Skinner, in the 1940's, elaborated on the powerful effects of reward by modifying behavior in pigeons.

These and other learning theorists are ideologically at odds with the followers of Sigmund Freud, who hold that unconscious thoughts and desires govern behavior. Their conclusions are based more often on introspection (what is true of me must be true of others) and observation of individuals undergoing treatment for emotional disturbance. The learning theorists, or behaviorists, have often overclaimed the power of their techniques. John Watson boasted that he could shape the behavior of a child almost at will. However, the learning theorists do have experimental evidence to show that human beings behave, at least with regard to automatic behavior, according to the principles of learning theory. On the other side, the very nature of the theories of the Freudians and psychologists of other "unconscious" schools does not permit the marshaling of a significant amount of experimental data showing the efficacy of their therapy.

To many acquainted with the Freudian tradition—nearly everybody, inasmuch as Freudian ideas have penetrated education, literature, and even journalism—the learning-theory techniques of behavior change often seem too cold, too mechanistic, and too animalistic. The systematic application of self-reward and self-punishment sounds self-conscious and silly because it does not get at the why of the behavior. But I believe that the two theories are not mutually exclusive. Unless a person has some insight into his behavior beyond that of understanding stimulus-response, he may not be able to develop enough general motivation to carry through on the details. Then, too, one needs to understand which stimuli produce which trains of behavior. Since so many stimuli are emotional, that is, responses to other human beings, understanding emotional psychology will help make easier the identification of stimuli for automatic behavior.

In defense of learning theory, there are at least three points to be made, in addition to its substantial scientific underpinnings.

The first is that, in attempting to form or to change everyday habits, we are dealing with the surface characteristics of our lives. Would anyone seriously argue that we must understand the psychological reason for tying shoelaces before we acquired the habit of doing so? Is the psychological "why" (in Freudian terms) important in switching from beef to fish? I cannot find any evidence that it is. Even if, in some particular case, fish had a negative psychological connotation and the reason was understood, there would still be the problem of switching. In any case, other methods of habit formation also use techniques of learning theory, but in a much less systematic way. The injunction to repeat an act many times if you want to form a habit is merely an attempt to create high-frequency behavior without using the power of reward.

The second point is that while the learning theory of habit formation rests on animal experiments, there are human data to confirm the animal findings. Nevertheless, we should not hide from our animal nature—nor can we. It is better to take advantage of it, control it for our benefit. Besides, I am not saying that all our behavior should or can be governed by learning theory, although some psychologists have made the claim. There is an ingredient in human behavior that is random, creative, unpredictable, and nonautomatic, perhaps even Freudian. I am only suggesting that we use learning theory to govern those aspects of our lives that are and should be automatic and thoughtless, our habits.

Finally, growing scientific evidence links the reward/punishment principle to drug addiction. It provides an important theoretical framework for understanding addictions and preventing them. Remember, I am not dealing with sick people—the cure of the addict is beyond the scope of this book. I am trying to show that it is possible to intervene at an early stage and change habits, long before they become irreversible, by the simple self-reward and self-punishment technique.

The reward/punishment scheme has another advantage. Most people who want to change their diet or cut back on smoking or drinking understand the deleterious effects of excesses. Nevertheless, though often well motivated to start making changes, they simply have quit after a while: "I've tried but I cannot continue." Usually, years of reward following undesired behavior have so firmly established the bad habit that a simple desire to change is not enough to break that habit. By systematizing rewards and punishments for habit change, you have the best chance of building motivation for the new habit as you go along. It is at least worth a try.

3 / To Work Harder Easier

It is not enough to be smart. You have to know how to work and work consistently. How often have you seen somebody who is not as intelligent as you seem to get ahead faster than you simply because he knows how to "buckle down" (barring the fact that his brother-in-law may own the business), while you hardly tap a tenth of your potential? At the same time, you find yourself (only from time to time, it is hoped) hating what you must do: reports, taking care of customers, passing civil-service exams, checking forms, or, if you work at home, taking care of the house, the laundry, the cooking, the beds, the sweeping, the garden. It is "hateful" and "boring." Each day, at home or at work, you start out with good intentions, but you quickly find your mind wandering. At the office, you can hardly wait for the coffee break. You get on the telephone. You quit early for lunch. At home, you read a book, a newspaper, a magazine; you sleep late, telephone friends, get away from the house. Everything except getting down to the work.

Work habits—good ones or bad—thus have a profound effect on your life. They can even affect your health by interacting with your eating, exercise, and smoking habits. This chapter deals with changing work habits; I put it here even though they are not as crucial to your health as diet, exercise, smoking, drinking, and the rest, because changing work habits is easier to comprehend and to accomplish. If you understand this chapter, you will find the others easier.

Obviously, poor work habits can have quite punishing results. Just to name a few, in order of increasing disaster:

- You may not like working or the work you have to do.
- You may find yourself not liking your home or your place of employment.
- You may earn less money.
- You may not get ahead in your career or job or school.
- Your cohabitant may not like living with you.
- You may hate your job or homework or school.
- You may be demoted at work or school.
- You may lose your job—quit or be fired.
- Your cohabitant may hate you, leading perhaps to a breakup.
- You may feel your entire life is worthless and pointless.

Given the fact that you must work, either at home, school, or job, it would be better if you could avoid all these consequences. And you can, simply by changing your work habits. That's all they are—habits. With improved work habits, you can do more in less time. But beyond that, you can win for yourself the following prizes:

- You can get to like (possibly even love) your work, school, home, place of employment.
- You can earn more money, get better grades, perhaps even live longer (by working more safely), and get ahead in your job.
- You can improve your interpersonal relations at work and at home.

Fortunately, behavioral science has developed techniques that you can apply to changing your work habits. These behavior-modification methods work, provided your bad work habits are not entrenched in a deep-seated mental disturbance. (If they are, you may need to work with a behavior therapist to help you change those habits.)

Studying

Since nearly everybody has been to school and has had to study, I will start with the example of studying as a work habit in order to describe how behavior-modification techniques are applied for change.

Let's start with the purpose of studying. You study a book or other material in order to acquire new or understand old information; you can pass it on and also generate new information for yourself. You do not study to learn a skill; you cannot learn to type simply by reading a book: you must type. Study is distinct from skill mastery, which we will discuss later.

As far back as 1946, scientists identified the important ingredients of good study habits. They called it the Survey Q3R technique. Q3R stands for *question, read, recite,* and *review.* Each word stands for a different behavior, which, if carried out correctly, contributes to your retention of information, your ability to understand it, and your ability to use it. I have never had any difficulty in studying or absorbing large amounts of material from books and magazines, and it was only in preparation for this book and my review of the scientific literature that I learned I had been using the Survey Q3R technique all my life. In college, I never took notes in lectures, nor did I underline my texts or take notes from them. Even today, as a reporter, I take few notes. My whole drive has been to understand the material and to be able to absorb it. And it is in this that I used, unknowingly, Survey Q3R. I had magnificent results from it (I won't brag about my college grades), and was thus rewarded promptly; so I continued to use it. Let me describe it a little more fully.

SURVEY. You begin by doing a quick survey of the material. If the book has boldface headings over the sections, you read them. If not, you read random first sentences of paragraphs throughout the section you are about to study. At the beginning of each school term, I used to sit down with all my texts, read all the tables of contents, and then read randomly within each text, skipping things I didn't understand. As you can see, *survey* gives you an overall view of the material. Then, as you subsequently read through it, you are able to readily grasp specific ideas because the general scope of the work is already familiar to you as a result of your preliminary survey: it is as if you had set up a coat rack in your brain and then hung the coats (the ideas) on it later. *Survey* should proceed at the rate of about five minutes for every fifty pages of text.

QUESTION. In this phase you ask yourself questions about the basic ideas you have picked up in your survey. It is a good idea to formulate the questions during a second scan of the basic headings. Ask the questions in your head. I used to jot down key words, about three or four of them, on a piece of paper that I intended to throw away. These were not notes, simply little reminders during the study period. Spend two minutes on *question* for every fifty pages of text.

READ. Next, read as fast as you can, trying to answer the questions that you raised during the question phase. Don't worry about not completely understanding what you are reading. Read the whole section you intended to read and then go back to reread the parts you didn't quite grasp. DO NOT UNDERLINE THE TEXT. DO NOT TAKE NOTES. JUST READ. If you underline or take notes, then you will focus on those behaviors and not on reading and answering the questions you raised for yourself. If you have been underlining and taking notes during reading, you are expending effort for a low return and you will not efficiently absorb or understand the material.

RECITE. This is the most critical behavior in studying. It means being able to reproduce, outline, or otherwise "recite" the information you have just read, without looking at the book. In studying geometry, I used to see if I could prove the propositions without referring to the book. I still retain large chunks of geometry.

There are several methods of reciting. You can outline what you have just read in a notebook, if your instructor requires one, or on a piece of paper—and then throw it away (that takes guts; I used to do it all the time, and I found I didn't need the paper). During a lecture, do not take notes (that, too, takes guts); outline the material afterward. You can write a little essay about it—and have the added benefit of writing practice at the same time. Or you can simply recite the material out loud, if you are in a place where people won't mind; if you are lucky enough to have a tape recorder, you can recite into it. The point is that in some way you must regurgitate what you have read or listened to without referring to the book or notes.

One way to avoid using the book is to sit on it; another is to toss it across the room, out of reach. Whatever you do, don't look at it while you are in the *recite* phase. Do not worry about omissions or errors. You take care of that with the third R.

REVIEW. After you have finished your recitation, check it

against an outline of the material in the book (by chapter headings or the like).

Now, all of this sounds like a lot of work. You think, If I do all that, I'll go twice as slowly as I did before. You will—in the beginning. But you will more than make up the time because you will practically eliminate the necessity of extensive reviewing and cramming later. And as you get the technique to the point where it is a habit, you will find, as I did, that the whole process goes much more quickly than reading and either simultaneously taking notes or underlining, both of which are inferior to Survey Q3R.

The Behavior Problem

Although it is easy enough to understand the technique—the scheme is simple—the problem lies in *doing* it, just as is the case with changing eating or exercise habits. Scientists who have studied Survey Q3R find that most students rather easily grasp and carry out *survey, question,* and *read. Recite* is the block. Reading is a familiar and relatively easy activity; but recitation requires a new kind of effort: remembering things and putting them together, composing. It is a new behavior to be learned through applying behavior-modification techniques. These techniques will also remedy any trouble you might have with *survey, question,* or even *read.*

Why do people have trouble studying? Teachers most often point to lack of motivation. That may be true enough. But where does that leave the student? How can he build motivation? A reward presented long after the desired behavior has less effect than a reward that comes immediately afterward. Thus the promise of high grades or monetary benefit is relatively ineffectual in the face of the punishing effort that a student has to make to absorb material that is difficult and possibly of only marginal interest. Some students can keep the image of higher grades or a "pay-off" before them constantly; the image thus acts as a thought reward following study. I have a hunch, however, that such students have learned the Survey Q3R technique and can easily connect their current studying with future reward. Study simply is not that hard for them.

Another problem is that the student finds his mind wandering. He puts the book down and seeks a diversion: food, telephoning a friend, daydreaming. His concentration on the book is fitful at best.

The student often encounters a third problem: the amount to be learned piles up if study is neglected early on. The sheer bulk of work is so threatening that it becomes punishing—and punishment, or the threat of it, will deter behavior. We all are familiar enough with the tendency to put off onerous work.

But let's examine some of the behavioral methods one can use to deal with the three major problems of study.

STIMULUS CONTROL. Fortunately, a large part of our behavior is automatic response to signals—stimuli—around us. But this automatic-response behavior can seriously interfere with the attempt to study, especially if that attempt is made without concern for the location. The sights and sounds of a cafeteria, for instance, or of a living room, can trigger automatic—and distracting—thoughts.

In order to control that stimulus-response, confine your studying to a particular time and place. In fact, it works even better if you study one subject at one time and place, and pick another time and place for another subject. At school, select a quiet alcove in the library with nobody else around. Study halls have many and various stimuli; they absolutely kill studying for people who have trouble with it. At home, use the same chair and the same corner of the room. If you have a desk, use it only for study. Do your letter-writing, bill-paying, telephoning somewhere else. A writer friend of mine used to write at home but found that the only way he could acquire stimulus control was to take an office downtown. I find that I have better luck with writing lately when I confine it to my desk at the same time every day. I do all other desk activities elsewhere in the house.

Once you have decided on your time and place, you proceed to bring yourself under control within that situation. Suppose you are studying history for the first time in your newly chosen specific location. You are in the *read* phase of Survey Q3R. And then your mind begins to wander and you cannot concentrate on the book. Do three things:

• Make up your mind to leave and quit studying.

• Read one more page in the book.
• After you have read the page, leave—even though your interest has revived.

Thus you have taken action to prevent your chosen location from becoming a stimulus for daydreaming. Do not return until the next day at the same time. Go do anything you like; do not punish yourself for leaving.

Well, you say, I won't get much done that way. I'll be leaving after three minutes every day! And besides, I have to get that assignment done tomorrow. What to do? Proceed to the next behavior-control technique.

SELF-MONITORING. One of the most important ingredients in behavior control is monitoring—either by counting the number of times you perform the desired behavior or measuring the time that behavior was sustained. This tells you whether you are carrying out the behavior as often as necessary in order to make it a habit.

The easiest way to do this is to make a simple chart with graph paper; if you don't have any, you can make your own with a ruler. I know it all sounds somewhat mechanical, but it is really the best way of keeping track of what you are doing. After you have the habit going, you can throw the chart away.

Suppose that in order to keep up with the required amount of history reading, you must establish a reading rate of forty pages an hour with the full Survey Q3R method. At the beginning of establishing stimulus control, you find that you read only five pages before you have to leave because of mind-wandering. You simply set a realistic goal; for instance, every day you will read about a page more than you did the day before. If the material is very difficult, set the increment lower. If you read more than your goal before your mind wanders and you have to leave, fine. After a month your graph should look something like the one on page 43. Across the bottom are the number of days of studying; the vertical simply records the number of pages read per day.

As the sample graph shows, there will be days on which you may not achieve your goal; you will drop back. That is okay. Just try the next day to meet the goal of one page more. At some point you will notice that your achievement rate accelerates. Eventu-

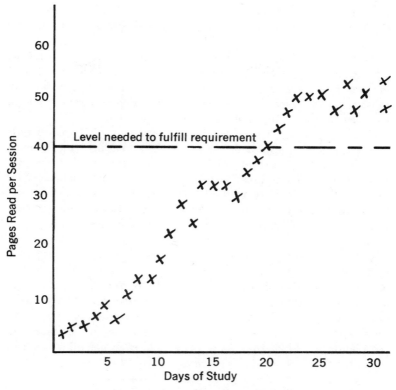

A Self-Monitoring Chart for Reading

ally, if you have set a realistic goal (if forty pages is too high for you, set it lower), you will probably go over it, because your skill will have improved and the habit will be reinforced.

You can use such self-monitoring charts for any behavior—to record the time it takes you to clean a room, for instance, if you have a tendency to dawdle (in that case the graph will show a declining curve). To do any kind of timing, you should use a stop watch. You can get one for about ten dollars. It's much cheaper than a vacuum cleaner and more than worth the price if you can reduce your cleaning time.

Self-monitoring charts can also be helpful in learning all the behaviors of the Survey Q3R method. As I mentioned, most students have trouble with *recite;* many with *question;* a few with *review.*

APPROXIMATION. No athlete breaks a record the first time he tries a particular sport. No student reads French at a glance if he has never seen the language before. There is a training and learning period in which small steps are taken before large. Thus, in learning to study, you should start with small steps.

Suppose you are having trouble with *question.* You can decide to do only one question for each boldface heading (or for each first sentence). Example: the heading for this section is "Approximation." What question could one ask? A simple one would be: What does it mean in the context of behavior modification? Or, another: How does he know it will work? But confine yourself to one question. The next day, try two questions per heading, and so on.

After you have mastered the first three steps and are ready for *recite,* try it one section at a time. Suppose you used this section. You would read it through, close the book and sit on it, try to answer the questions you had raised after *survey,* and then either outline it, write a short essay, or talk it into a recorder. Your self-monitoring chart can keep track of the number of sections you read before reciting. But you approximate each behavior in small steps. *Do not do more than you can do comfortably.*

REWARDS. There are several kinds of rewards you can use to reinforce desired behavior. A self-monitoring chart is one rewarding mechanism: you see tangible results immediately after performing the behavior. For many people just observing their abilities climb is strongly reinforcing. However, you must discover what is powerful enough for you.

I have a self-reward trick that I use when I am writing a long article or chapter in a book. I like iced tea (in winter, hot tea). At my desk I set up a Thermos (cost: under three dollars, cheaper than a book). Then I flip a coin and, without looking at it, place it under the Thermos. (Remember that if you start out rewarding your new behavior *every* time, that behavior will be difficult to sustain when inevitably there is no reward present. Random rewards are more powerful reinforcers in the long run.)

After completing a page of manuscript, I lift the flask. If it's heads up, I take a couple of swallows of tea; if it's tails, I don't and get on with the next page. That serves two purposes: I get random rewards and I do not drink too much tea. (I use a version of this technique to get up in the morning, too.)

You can use coffee, low-calorie soft drinks, or anything you like in order to time the completion of a set amount of work. Now, if you decide to check the coin every time you've read a page—about every minute or so—in an hour you will rate about thirty rewards, which may be more tea or soda pop than you want to drink. In that case, shake up two coins and put them under the Thermos. Drink only if both are heads. That will cut your reward frequency down to about fifteen an hour, and if you take only a mouthful each time, you will keep your liquid intake normal. You could reward yourself after two pages, but if you are trying to develop a habit, frequent reinforcement works better. It may be that you will have to set the reward schedule for after every half page or paragraph. Set your own pace—whatever works better for you and keeps your liquid intake modest. If you overdo it, the drink will lose its reward power.

Remember that thought rewards can be used, too: the anticipation of passing a test, a higher grade, a better job, the approval of the teacher or other students . . . anything you find pleasant and desirable. However, do not dawdle too long on the pleasant scene: it leads to daydreaming. A good way to cut off the scene is to use the stop-thought technique discussed in the next chapter. It can also be used if you find yourself daydreaming: try the stop-thought method once. If it doesn't work, abandon it and go through the quitting procedure.

Skill Mastery

The study-behavior skills of Survey Q3R can be mastered in the same way you master other skills: typing, piano-playing, arithmetic, writing, spelling . . . you name it. The essential factor in skill mastery is practice, as anybody could guess. But admonitions to practice are as plentiful as help in organizing it is rare.

The same behavior-control methods described in learning to study can facilitate practice enormously: stimulus control, self-monitoring, and reward. An additional method, implicit in the study-behavior technique, is repetition of the *same* behavior. Typing affords a good example: you can increase your speed in typing by retyping the same sentences several times rather than by constantly typing new material.

I do not say that just by using behavior-control methods you will become a champion typist or a fantastic musician or a marvelous writer. For any of those achievements, you also need indefinable talent, drive, and other qualities. But you can become efficient enough in these and other skills so that they are useful to you at home and at your job; and you can learn them more quickly and with less psychic effort.

Let's go back to the typing example. Get a typing practice manual, then pick a time and place that will provide stimulus control. On the first day establish how much you can do before your mind wanders or you get tired or uncomfortable. Construct a self-monitoring chart and record the number of lines typed before you quit. Set up a system of random rewards, as discussed before, and use them after a set number of lines has been typed.

When you make up your mind to quit, type a few more lines—the number of which you have established beforehand—and then quit. Do not go back even though you feel encouraged to.

When you return the next time, retype about half of what you did the last time and go on from there. Each day increase the quota of typing by a small fixed amount, not so much as to make yourself uncomfortable, but more than you did the day before. However, even if you have not reached that goal by the time your mind starts to wander or you get upset or tired, quit.

After you have mastered most of the keys, start timing your efforts. Use a self-monitoring chart in which the goal is now words per minute as well as lines typed. Again, start at a low level and slowly build up speed. In developing speed, it is important that you practice the same passage at least three times. Reward yourself after each passage; record your progress; quit if you feel uncomfortable (but only after you attempt one more trial).

Other skills can be mastered in the same way. The secret of

learning to write is to rewrite your material twice and three times—it is then that rewarding systems and stimulus control are very useful. I find that reading good writing has improved my writing; perhaps listening to good music does the same for musicians. In both cases, a skilled individual is providing a model for you to follow. It is my belief that teachers are more important for the kind of model they are to the student than for the information or skills they impart.

Chores

The housekeeper's lament that there is never enough time usually succumbs to good behavior-modification plans. Performing chores with speed and efficiency leaves plenty of time to do those things that are more profitable, emotionally as well as economically. How are efficient chore habits developed?

Chores present a slightly different problem than studying or skill mastery because stimulus control does not come as readily: you must be in many different places around the house or apartment and you must perform many different behaviors in a single place. However, self-monitoring still helps, particularly if you work against time. Make a self-monitoring chart for putting a room in order (see page 48).

Time yourself with a stop watch and resolve to speed up your time by, say, fifteen seconds each day. Make the decrement small enough to be comfortable for you. After a number of days or weeks, you will reach a plateau.

If you have trouble at the beginning decreasing the time, you may be having stimulus-control or reward problems. In that case, make a self-monitoring chart similar to the pages-read chart and follow the instructions for creating a stimulus-control situation. Example: you start to tidy up your bedroom; the stop watch is going. At the point when you feel your mind wandering away from the job and you find yourself just standing there daydreaming, or you are getting frustrated and uncomfortable, make up your mind to quit after you do, say, thirty seconds more work. Do not continue, even though you feel encouraged to do more. Leave the bed unmade, or whatever. Do not return to it later on; leave it

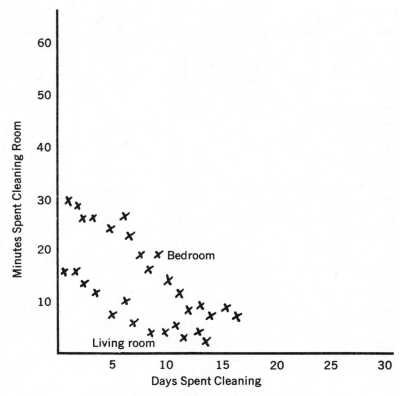

A Self-Monitoring Chart for Room-Cleaning

for the next day. But do record how much time you spent tidying up. Each day you should try to spend *more* time on whatever chore needs doing. Finally, after a few days, you will find yourself completing the job of tidying and your graph will grow just like the pages-read chart. After you have achieved job completion, make a second self-monitoring room-cleaning chart to speed up your work.

You can use the rewards of soft drink, tea, coffee, or whatever appeals to you after the completion of a segment of the job—after you have made the bed, say, or after you have swept the floor, picked up the newspapers, et cetera. Don't forget to use the random-reward system.

Premack's Principle

There is another form of reward that can be very effective in managing chores. You are familiar with it as the second law of behavior. It is known as "Premack's Principle" (after Dr. David Premack, who formulated it): any activity or behavior can be a reward for another behavior. The rewarding behavior must be more frequent than the rewarded behavior. Suppose, for example, that every morning you automatically pick up the newspapers scattered around the bedroom from the night before. That habit is a frequent behavior. If you now deliberately start out by first making the bed and then picking up the papers, the latter will act as a reward for having made the bed.

I used Premack's Principle to keep my desk at the office relatively neat: whenever the phone rang, I first put one piece of paper in place (the infrequent behavior) and then answered the telephone (the frequent behavior). You can use the technique in learning to fasten your safety belt: do it before you turn the ignition key or before you close the car door. As you can see, this system can be readily introduced in all kinds of work or activity problems. Just do the *uncomfortable* work before you do the *comfortable*. You will not be decreasing the instances of frequent behavior, but rather increasing the instances of infrequent behavior. Do the rotten job first; reward yourself with the good job.

Summary

Remember the sequence of behavior control: analyze the job (it takes five minutes); set up self-monitoring charts; establish some sort of reward mechanism, either material rewards, like soft drinks, or thought rewards, or by applying Premack's Principle; establish stimulus control by confining the work to one place and time.

As you learn the technique, you will find it easier and easier to modify those old, inefficient habits and replace them with more efficient ones. Skill mastery will be a less onerous chore. You will find you have more time for pleasurable activities—and after a while you may even find that the required work is fun to do.

4 / Relax and Change Your Life Style

When I first went to work as a broadcaster, I discovered that if I were to succeed at my new job, it would be necessary to part with a way of speaking that had been with me all of my life. My Brooklyn-born-and-bred singsong would have to be replaced by a deep-voiced delivery of clearly pronounced consonants and non-nasal vowels.

Learning to speak in a new way was not too much of a problem, thanks to a speech coach. Psychologically, it was quite a different story: I found that I harbored a fear of changing my lifelong habit of speech. Wouldn't my friends make fun of me? Wouldn't they think I was putting on airs? To my ears, my new speech sounded awful. I was losing something I had always thought was the *real* me. This new-talking man was somebody else.

I wish I had known in 1966 that there is a method of changing lifelong habits and simultaneously reducing such fears. If I had realized that the real me was the me I *chose* to be, forming the new habit would have been much less painful. That method of reducing fear and speeding up habit change involves physical relaxation.

Relaxation as a Tool

Although people have been enjoying the benefits of physical relaxation for centuries, it was not scientifically scrutinized until the 1930's. Edmund Jacobson, a Chicago physician, developed an elaborate ritual for first relaxing groups of muscles and then measuring the degree of relaxation electrically. His patients had difficulty in learning to relax; sometimes Dr. Jacobson would have to work on one little group of muscles for days. But he was motivated by his belief that much psychic tension—what is now called "anxiety"—arose from the inability to relax.

What causes psychic tension, or anxiety? Countless situations arise every day that can, to a greater or lesser degree, cause anxiety: pressure on the job, difficulties at home, health or money crises. Ordinarily, the body's response to mental stress is muscle tension. Even after the initial stimulus for the psychic anxiety recedes, the muscles remain tensed—with the result that you feel tired, have aches and pains in your back, neck, arms, and face, look strained, and have difficulty sleeping.

To counter these annoying symptoms, that is, to relax, many people resort to alcohol, cigarettes, or food. Popping pills has, unfortunately, joined the ranks of favorite relaxants. But, as a number of studies show, turning to drugs or food rather than turning to people or activities for relaxation brings only temporary relief. More important, alcohol, cigarettes, food, and pills carry the risks of ill health and addiction.

Dr. Jacobson showed that a person can be trained to relax. Just as you can learn to type or to speak a foreign language, so you can learn a relaxation technique. Once learned, it can be invoked instantly—in the time it takes to light a cigarette, take a drink or a pill, or eat a chocolate bar.

Relaxation as a means of controlling psychic tension will be the burden of our discussion here. But it has many other applications. A West German physician, Dr. J. H. Schultz, has for years prescribed his own brand of relaxation for a variety of ills, from asthma to schizophrenia. Unfortunately, his claims for "autogenic training," as he calls it, are not backed up by substantial scientific evidence. And transcendental meditation, in which the participant is trained to concentrate on an interior sound, creates relaxation, as does hypnosis.

All relaxation techniques produce similar physical responses: lowered heart rate, slower breathing, muscular relaxation, and even chemical changes in the blood. I confess I could hardly believe that transcendental meditation had any value until I saw the scientific data. I am still somewhat doubtful of claims that relaxation methods can make enormous changes in an individual's life style. But relaxation can be a great help; of that I am sure. For example:

Dr. Joseph Wolpe is a psychiatrist who applies behavior-modification techniques to the treatment of neurosis. His theory is that if he can produce in the patient a response—relaxation— antagonistic to anxiety in the presence of a stimulus that provokes anxiety, the connection between the anxiety and the stimulus will be weakened.

Suppose a man feels desperately anxious every time a dog comes near him. If he can be made to relax—which is antagonistic to anxiety—when he is near a dog, he will feel less anxious the next time a dog approaches. The man thus feels rewarded by the reduction of his anxiety and the desired behavior—relaxation in the presence of the anxiety stimulus—is reinforced. Evidence that such a method can cure phobias has been well established scientifically; there is less evidence that neurosis can be thus eliminated, although Dr. Wolpe and others have impressive records.

In Dr. Wolpe's technique the patient is first taught to relax through a shortened version of the Jacobson method. While in the relaxed state, the patient is asked to conjure up a pleasant scene, which of course is different for different people. If he cannot picture a particular scene, he is told to try to visualize the word calm.

Next, patient and therapist draw up a list of anxiety-provoking mental images in order of increasing potency. For the man who is made anxious by a dog, the list might be:

1. A furry animal
2. The word dog
3. A specific image of a dog
4. The dog approaching the patient
5. The dog standing three feet away

6. The dog right next to him
7. The patient allowing the dog to nuzzle him
8. The patient petting the dog

In the third step in Dr. Wolpe's technique the therapist asks the patient to think of the first image on the list. The therapist might say:

"Now that you are relaxed, think of that pleasant scene—the one where you're at the beach—and just relax all your muscles. Now, as you're relaxing, you see in the distance a little furry animal [a three-second pause]. Stop imagining the furry animal . . . think only of relaxing your muscles . . . and again, now, of the pleasant scene [a ten-second pause]. If the thought of that little furry animal bothers you at all, just raise your index finger a little. [If the patient raises his finger, he is told to stop imagining the furry-animal scene.] If not, just keep thinking about the little furry animal way off in the distance on that beach. . . ."

The therapist goes through each image on the list in the same way, until the patient no longer feels anxiety about it. Some therapists actually bring the feared objects into the patient's presence during the relaxation sessions.

In terms of our reward/punishment scheme, the pleasant scene and the relaxation act as rewards for the patient's learning the new behavior of not feeling anxious in the presence of a particular stimulus. Dr. Wolpe would put it another way: the state of relaxation and the pleasant mental image in the presence of the offending stimulus weaken the power of the stimulus to provoke anxiety.

This method, which goes by various names, including "desensitization" and "reciprocal inhibition," has been used successfully by therapists. There is no evidence, however, that an individual can, without the help of a therapist, cure himself of deep-seated phobias and neuroses. But there is evidence that the development of the ability to relax and to imagine both pleasant and punishing scenes can be a useful tool in changing habits. If you are a normal person with normal problems, you can employ the method to advantage: in diet control, in an exercise program—if you have fears that you will be in some way injured by the hard exercise you are doing—or in a stop-smoking campaign. You can relax, imagine a fear—say of pulling a muscle—and try to stay relaxed while thinking of the fear. If you cannot sustain relaxation, use a less-feared consequence, working your way gradually to the most potent.

Stopping Your Thoughts

To make full use of the relaxation technique to change your habits, you also need another skill: stopping thoughts. Actually, it is quite simple. If you have a thought that bothers you, you can stop it by shouting out loud or imagining yourself shouting Stop! Try it. Think of something. Anything. Then shout, Stop! You will find that that thought momentarily clears away. And if you take advantage of that moment, you can turn your thoughts to some other scene. Thought-stopping is useful also in cutting off unwanted daydreams, or as an aid to stopping those nighttime thoughts that keep you awake. You will hear more about thought-stopping in this book.

Relaxing

You can learn to relax by listening to recorded instructions. Dr. Herbert Fensterheim, a behavior therapist, included a transcript of such a recording in his book *Help Without Psychoanalysis.** I present it here as one of the clearest versions of several I have seen. If you have a tape recorder, have a friend read the passage into it. (Of course, you can do it yourself if your own voice doesn't bother you.) If possible, the reader should have a deep, soothing voice. The parts that instruct you to tense up should be read sharply; those that bid you relax should be read slowly, mellifluously, almost bordering on the hypnotic. Find a comfortable bed or couch, or use the floor with a rug on it.

The whole process takes seventeen minutes. After you have been successful with this version, you can proceed to a shorter version that you create yourself. The end result will be that you can relax in a moment, almost no matter where you are, by simply recalling the instructions, or just by holding your breath for a few seconds and then exhaling.

---

* New York: Stein and Day, 1971. Used with permission.

The 17-Minute Relaxation Instruction

Lie down. Your eyes are closed. Your arms are at your sides, your fingers open. Get yourself good and comfortable. If stray thoughts enter your mind, say to yourself, Stop! Push them away and concentrate on what we are doing. . . . (A) The first thing to do is tighten the muscles in the lower part of your body. Turn your feet inward, pigeon-toed, heels slightly apart. Curl your toes tightly, bend your feet downward away from you . . . now upward toward you . . . this tightens the muscles along your shins and in your calves . . . at the same time tighten up your thighs, tighten up the muscles of your buttocks, and the muscles around your anus . . . not so tight that they are strained, but tight enough to feel the tension . . . study it, study the tension . . . tense, tense, tense . . . (*five-second pause*)

Now relax . . . just feel the tension flow out . . . concentrate on relaxing the muscles of your toes . . . relax the muscles of your legs . . . relax the muscles of your thighs . . . relax your buttocks, the muscles around your anus . . . now concentrate on each part of your body as I name it . . . toes relaxed . . . legs relaxed . . . thighs relaxed . . . muscles of your buttocks . . . relaxed . . . all the tension out . . . (*ten-second pause*)

Now tighten up the muscles of your abdomen. Make the muscles of your abdomen as taut as if a child were going to shove a football into your stomach . . . get them good and tight . . . study the tension . . . feel where the tension is . . . hold it for ten seconds . . . hold it . . . tense . . . tense . . . tense. . . .

And now relax . . . relax the muscles of your abdomen . . . let them go . . . try to relax the muscles deep inside your abdomen . . . the muscles of your gut . . . let them go . . . you are more and more relaxed . . . (*ten-second pause*)

And now the muscles of your back . . . arch your back . . . arch the small of your back until you feel the tension build . . . try to locate the tension . . . there are two long muscle columns alongside your spine . . . you may feel the tension there . . . wherever it is get to know the feel of tension . . . your back is tense . . . tense . . . tense. . . .

And now relax . . . relax the muscles of your back . . . let them go . . . let all the tension out . . . your back feels limp and heavy . . . let it stay that way . . . more and more relaxed . . . (*ten-second pause*)

And now the muscles of your chest . . . take a deep breath and hold it . . . just keep on holding it . . . five seconds . . . notice as you hold your breath the tension begins to build up . . . note the tension in your chest muscles . . . study where it is . . . ten seconds . . . keep holding your breath . . . recognize the feeling of tension . . . fifteen seconds . . . now slowly, as slowly as you can . . . let your breath out . . . slowly . . . now breathe easily and comfortably, as in a deep sleep . . . (*pause*) . . . keep on relaxing the muscles of your chest . . . let them go . . . let the tension out . . . (*ten-second pause*)

Now concentrate on each part as I mention it . . . abdomen relaxed . . . back relaxed . . . chest relaxed . . . all the tension out . . . (*pause*)

And now the muscles of your fingers, arms, and shoulders . . . make a tight fist with each hand . . . keep your elbows stiff and straight as rods . . . raise your arms from the shoulders to a forty-five-degree angle . . . the angle of your arms is halfway between the couch and the vertical . . . now feel the tension . . . study the tension . . . study the tension in your fingers . . . in your forearms . . . in your arms and your shoulders . . . hold the tension for ten seconds . . . hold it . . . hold it . . . tense . . . tense . . . tense. . . .

And now relax . . . fingers open . . . arms down to sides . . . just relax . . . relax the muscles of your fingers . . . of your forearms . . . let them go . . . relax the muscles of your upper arms . . . let them go . . . and now the muscles of your shoulders . . . let them go . . . (*pause*) . . . fingers relaxed . . . arms relaxed . . .

shoulders relaxed . . . let your arms feel limp and heavy . . . just keep letting go . . . (*ten-second pause*)

And now the muscles between the shoulder blades and the muscles of your neck . . . pull your shoulders back until your shoulder blades are almost touching . . . at the same time arch your neck until your chin points at the ceiling . . . these are areas very sensitive to nervous tension . . . many people feel most of their tension here . . . feel the tension . . . not so tight that it hurts . . . study the tension . . . let it build up . . . (*ten-second pause*)

Now relax . . . relax the muscles between your shoulder blades . . . let the tension flow out . . . let it go . . . and relax the muscles of your neck . . . let them go . . . your neck muscles are not supporting your head . . . your head is limply falling against the pillow . . . all the tension out . . . feel it flowing out . . . (*thirty-second pause*)

And now the muscles of the upper part of your face . . . make a grimace with the top part of your face . . . squeeze your eyes tight shut . . . wrinkle your nose . . . frown . . . notice where you feel the tension . . . study it . . . note that you feel the tension in the forehead, between the eyebrows, in the cheeks below the eyes. . . .

Now relax . . . let all the tension out . . . just concentrate on relaxing the muscles of your forehead . . . let them go . . . relax your eyelids . . . as they relax you note they begin to feel heavy . . . they make you feel drowsy but you're not going to sleep . . . you must stay alert . . . relax the muscles at the bridge of your nose . . . let them go . . . relax the muscles of your cheeks . . . remember where they felt tight . . . let them go . . . (*ten-second pause*)

And now the muscles of your jaws and tongue . . . bite hard with your back teeth, press them together until your jaws are tight . . . feel the tension at your temples, by your ears . . . wherever you feel the tension, study it . . . push your tongue against the back of your lower front teeth . . . your jaws are tight . . . your tongue is tight . . . study the tension . . . get to know it . . . learn the feel of the tension . . . hold it, hold it . . . (*ten-second pause*)

Now relax . . . relax the muscles of your jaws . . . let them go . . . relax your tongue . . . your teeth should be slightly parted . . . your jaw is hanging slack . . . more and more relaxed . . . (*thirty-second pause*)

Now the muscles around the lower part of your face . . . tense the muscles around your mouth and chin . . . the best way to make them tense is to grin . . . a big grin, a grimace . . . draw back your lips to show your teeth, upper and lower teeth . . . draw the corners of your mouth wide, pull them back and down . . . feel the tension in your lips, around your mouth, in your chin . . . let the tension build up . . . hold it . . . feel it . . . study it . . . tense . . . tense . . . tense . . . (*ten-second pause*)

Now relax . . . relax the muscles around your mouth and chin . . . let them go . . . get all the tension out . . . (*thirty-second pause*). . . . Now try to relax the muscles of your throat . . . relax the soft part of your throat . . . relax the soft part of your throat where you swallow . . . relax the muscles of your voice box . . . just try to get all the tension out of there . . . (*thirty-second pause*)

That's the end of the first part of the exercise. . . . Keep your eyes closed; you're still relaxing.

Now for the second part. Just ask yourself: Is there any tension in my legs, in my thighs, in my buttocks? If there is, let it go . . . try to get all the tension out . . . more and more relaxed . . . (*ten-second pause*). . . . And now ask yourself: Is there any tension in my fingers, my arms, or my shoulders? . . . If there is, let it go . . . let your arms get limp and heavy . . . (*ten-second pause*). . . . Now ask yourself: Is there any tension between my shoulder blades or in my neck? . . . If there is, let it go . . . your head is falling limply back . . . (*pause*). . . . And now ask yourself: Is there any tension in my face, my jaws, or my throat? If there is, let it go . . . all the tension out . . . just keep letting go . . . (*pause*)

And now the third part of the exercise. Picture your pleasant scene or, if you have trouble with that picture, the word calm. . . . Get a good clear picture, not just the sight, but the sounds, the smells, and the feel . . . if your mind wanders, always bring it back to the pleasant scene. And while you hold that picture in mind, concentrate on relaxing the muscles of your toes . . . let them go . . . (*pause*) . . . relax the muscles of your thighs . . . let them go . . . (*pause*) . . . keep picturing that pleasant scene. If stray thoughts come into your mind, just tell yourself, Stop. Put them away. . . .

(B) [It is at this point that you can introduce the mental picture of the object about which you wish to change your attitude. Picture first the least disturbing idea. If it is too disturbing, stop the thought and go back to the pleasant scene and continue holding it in your mind and relaxing until you feel ready to try again. Try three times, or until you find the image not disturbing at all. If you experienced no disturbance just continue to relax until the end of the exercise and end with the pleasant scene again.]

Just concentrate on the muscles of your abdomen . . . let them go . . . relax . . . (*pause*). . . . Relax the muscles of your chest . . . breathe easily and comfortably . . . keep picturing your pleasant scene . . . (*pause*)

[You may try desensitization here.]

Relax the muscles of your fingers . . . let them go . . . (*pause*) . . . relax your forearms . . . (*pause*) . . . relax the muscles of your shoulders . . . let them go . . . (*pause*). . . . Keep picturing the pleasant scene. . . . Relax the muscles of your shoulder blades . . . let them go . . . (*pause*) . . . relax the muscles of your neck . . . let them go . . . (*pause*). . . . Keep the pleasant scene. . . . Relax the muscles of your forehead . . . let them go . . . (*pause*) . . . relax your eyelids . . . (*pause*) . . . relax the muscles at the bridge of your nose . . . let them go . . . (*pause*) . . . relax your jaw muscles . . . relax your tongue . . . relax the muscles around your mouth and chin . . . let them go . . . (*pause*) . . . relax the muscles of your throat . . . all the tension out . . .

let yourself feel limp and heavy all over. . . . Now keep
picturing the pleasant scene. . . .
[Another good place to try desensitization.]
    Calm and relaxed . . . calm and relaxed . . . (*ten-
second pause*). . . . If you feel tension anywhere, just let it
go . . . (*thirty-second pause*)
[You may try here again, but if it doesn't work, that is, if
you feel bothered by the scene, go back to your pleasant
scene and keep it in your imagination while relaxing for at
least thirty seconds before ending the relaxation as follows:]
    Now I'm going to count from three to one. At the count of
one you will sit up and open your eyes. You'll be alert and
wide awake and very refreshed . . . three . . . two . . .
one.

If you do try the desensitization procedure for changing your
attitudes toward food, exercise, or any other habit you wish to
change, please remember to continue relaxing if at any time your
mental picture bothers you. Before going on to picture your
pleasant scene again, use stop-thought to get the bothersome
image completely out of your mind. The stop-thought technique
enables you to banish disturbing thoughts from your mind for a
few seconds at first and later, with practice, for minutes and
hours.

To cut down the time of relaxation, simply shorten the periods
of relaxation of each group of muscles and eliminate everything
from section B on. In shortening the transcript it is only necessary to give the briefest of instruction. For example, the first
paragraph in section A could read: Curl your toes, tighten shins
and calves, thighs, anus and buttocks . . . hold for five seconds.
Now relax. . . . Relax legs . . . thighs . . . relax anus. . . .
Relax buttocks . . . (*ten-second pause*).

But do not proceed to a shortened version until after you have
learned to relax with the 17-Minute Instruction.

The Problem of Sleep

Millions of people have trouble getting to sleep. They lie awake
for what seems to be half the night, ruminating about the day's

events or past events, and are robbed of that sweet surcease, sleep. For untold numbers—probably millions—the solution is chemical: a barbiturate or some other kind of sleeping pill, or a shot of whisky. Unless they are under a physician's vigilance, these sleepless people find themselves taking more and more pills or more and more drink in trying to fall asleep. But modern sleep research suggests that chemically induced rest may deprive you of the kind of sleep that is most soothing and refreshing. Drugs disturb the normal cycle of dreaming, a cycle that appears to be related to waking behavior.

For millions of other people, the problem isn't so much getting to sleep as it is getting up in the morning. At least one study has established that, ironically, people who put in an extra hour or so of sleep end up with a worn-out feeling. Moreover, the oversleeping syndrome can also get you into trouble on the job, at school, and even at home. There are also many people for whom getting up is just as much of a problem as getting to sleep.

In general, sleep habits change with age. Older people go to sleep earlier and get up earlier. They tend to catch more naps during the day. Some people get along fine on four and a half hours of sleep; others are knocked out if they do not get ten. The average sleep time is seven and a half hours. Long sleepers apparently have a higher risk of death from a variety of diseases, though the connection is not well understood. It may be that long sleepers are those who use pills or alcohol to get to sleep and are thus vulnerable to the dangers of such measures.

Sleep as a Habit

In all the reading I've done about sleep, its habitlike characteristics stand out markedly. In *Sleep*, by Gay Gaer Luce and Dr. Julius Segal, the authors describe the ritual nature of many people's sleep habits: there are some children who need a certain blanket, adults who sleep in certain positions, many people who find it difficult to sleep in unfamiliar surroundings. Each of these situations is characterized by a stimulus-response mechanism— the blanket, the position, the familiar surroundings are all signals that start the chain of behavior leading to sleep.

If you have bad sleeping habits, you have to analyze what they are and then make use of a behavior-modification technique to change those habits. If you are in the habit of taking pills or alcohol to fall asleep, you will encounter serious difficulties in using behavior control. To stop resorting to these crutches means —as you well know—several nights of no sleep at all. It is the thought of this punishment that deters many people from seeking a natural way of getting to sleep. It is not impossible, however. You might consider enlisting the aid of a physician or a skilled behavior therapist to get you off medication, unless, of course, you are willing to put up with a few uncomfortable nights doing it on your own.

There are several things you can do to change from a bad sleep pattern to a good one. First, decide to go to sleep at the same time every night for several weeks, and to get up at the same time. At least one study shows that those persons who go to sleep at the same time every night have less difficulty in getting to sleep and rising. You should be in bed and ready for sleep at the chosen hour; don't be discouraged if for the first few nights—it may be as many as five—you don't get to sleep as soon as you would like.

Second, eat each meal at the same time every day; try to stick to that daily schedule. Studies done on people who have moved from one time zone to another indicate that those who keep to a strict daily schedule for meals and sleeping adjust most rapidly to the time change.

Third, have you thought of exercise? People who run, jog, cycle, or do some other form of activity regularly have less difficulty falling asleep than those who are sedentary. If you decide on an exercise program, however, do it at a time well before you go to bed. Physical activity just before bedtime can somewhat hinder sleep, although not nearly so much as intellectual activity. Heavy studying, card-playing, a heated conversation, or any other such mental exercise can make falling asleep difficult. For at least a half hour before bedtime, try doing all sorts of dull and trivial things. This will prevent the machinery of your brain from racing; consequently your mind will be more ready for sleep.

Fourth, check your bed. Is it comfortable? Most experts recommend a firm mattress. Check yours for lumps and sags. Your choice for a pillow.

Finally, master the relaxation instruction and go through it just before bedtime. You will be more likely to fall asleep quickly. That there is a connection between relaxation training and reduction of insomnia has clinical support. If your presleep ruminations seem to be uncontrollable, if you just cannot seem to get those thoughts out of your head, try adding the stop-thought technique to your relaxation program. You will then be focusing only on pleasant scenes; your tension level will decline and you will create a new set of stimuli for falling asleep.

A self-monitoring chart can be a useful guide to making any corrections in your sleep-change program. Keep track on a chart or a calendar of the number of nights on which you fall asleep quickly and the number you do not. Note what happens on the failure nights; perhaps you had a particularly exciting evening, or you failed to go to bed at your usual time or departed from your eating schedule. Maybe your exercise program is inconsistent. Keeping track of these minor breakdowns will help you to know just what your specific problems are so that you can be on guard against them.

Unfortunately, there is no study that demonstrates the total success of this program in solving sleep problems. However, given all the evidence pointing to a firm connection between relaxation and sleep, together with a strong suggestion that sleep has many characteristics of a habit, I feel safe in concluding that a behavior-modification program gives a normal person the best chance of solving a sleep problem. If your sleep is deeply disturbed, that is, if you get up after two or three hours and cannot go to sleep again, night after night, then something is seriously wrong. In such a case, it would be wise to consult a psychiatrist or behavior therapist.

Waking Up

If you regularize the times at which you go to sleep, then you will have less trouble waking up in the morning. About 30 per cent of the population has no trouble springing awake without the aid of an alarm of some kind; the other 70 per cent uses alarms. And alarms aren't always effective; many people merely turn the alarm off and roll over for an extra hour or so of sleep.

Waking up seems to be a habit, too. From the reward/punishment point of view, sleep can be preferable to facing the reality of the day—the home, the job, the world in general. Perhaps that reluctance is not on such a serious level for most of us; but we can all remember at least one instance where the pillow made a more attractive bid than the vacuum cleaner or the lawn mower, or the crowded subway on a rainy day.

A reward, even though apparently small, is more powerful if it immediately follows the desired behavior—which suggests that one way to solve the waking-up crunch is to reward yourself the minute you are conscious in the morning, and to continue to do so for remaining awake. Here is how it works for me: I set the alarm for the desired hour (the same each day). By the bedside I have a Thermos partially filled with cold fruit juice (it is a very good idea to vary the juice). Underneath the Thermos I keep a coin. Upon the ringing of the alarm, I get up, put my feet on the floor, and do not turn off the alarm until I have taken a sip of the cold juice. At first, I rewarded myself for each wake-up victory (standing up, starting to dress, et cetera). After a week, I started flipping the coin in order to give myself random rewards. Recall that random rewards reinforce a habit more strongly than rewards that always follow a desired behavior. It takes longer to create a habit with random reward but the habit holds up better in the absence of reward.

After a couple of weeks the habit seemed firm, and indeed proved so: one morning at the appointed hour I awakened and stayed awake in spite of the fact that I had forgotten to prepare the equipment and set the alarm the night before!

You might have trouble staying awake, resisting the temptation to go back to bed. If you like to drink coffee or tea in the morning, you might prepare two Thermos bottles, one with juice, one with coffee. To get your feet on the floor, use the juice; then reward yourself with your favorite hot drink for taking a shower (if you like, use the shower as a reward), getting dressed, or doing whatever is appropriate to a chain of behavior that will take you further and further away from the idea of bed.

Taking Advantage of Your Mind

Unlike nontalking, nonreading animals, we human beings have the power to manipulate symbols. We are also, to a greater extent than we like to believe, creatures of habit. As you will see, it is possible for us to put this manipulative power to work in order to change a habit, an attitude. No animal can do that. It is thoroughly human. Basically, *you* are in control.

5 / Moving to Stay Alive

Almost everyone believes that exercise is a good thing. Even if they are not aware of the extensive, though controversial, scientific evidence linking physical activity to protection against illness and shortened life, they can certainly appreciate the lithe, vibrant, good-looking bodies that exercise produces.

Perhaps you want to stop reading now because you feel guilty that the most exercise you get in a day is walking over to the dinner table. Please, don't feel bad. You have a lot of company. Only half the number of American adults exercise at all; the rest have sat down on the job of keeping their biological machinery in good working order. More than half the men and women who do take up some exercise program drop out; the record is as poor as that for diet-control projects. For the sedentary, exercise is a punishment, and punishment will kill a habit or prevent one from forming. When a sedentary person starts an exercise program, he usually does it in a way that hurts, really hurts.

According to the laws of habit formation, pain will prevent the formation of a habit unless that punishing pain is overridden by a powerful and *immediate* reward. There are many psychological experiments showing that both human beings and animals will prefer an easier task to one that requires physical effort, a common-sense discovery. However, contrary to popular belief, habits learned with effort die just as quickly as those learned without effort—which sort of explains why so many athletes quit exercising once they are no longer in competition. In some psychological tests, individuals who learned a habit by overcoming a physical-effort obstacle seemed to value the habit more than those who learned it the easy way. I guess that is the most one can say in favor of learning anything the hard way.

Our task here, then, is to remove the pain and punishment from exercise (it can be done) and to increase the immediate rewards for doing exercise. It will require a new way of thinking about behavior, a way that emphasizes how you do something, rather than why.

The Many Hopes of Exercise

It is discouraging to rummage through the vast scientific literature on exercise and physical activity only to discover endless reports on the efficacy of exercise in promoting health, on ways of throwing the javelin better, on motivational studies to teach young boys to jump higher . . . in short, everything you want to know about exercise, except the one thing you really want to know: how to start exercising and—how to keep on exercising.

Almost all the books and articles on the subject try to motivate Americans in a general way: exercise is good for you; it makes you look better, makes you feel better, psychologically and physically, because it cures or prevents all sorts of aches, pains, and terrible disease—all of which is more or less true. Such pep talks are designed to make you get out of the chair and start down the road on a program that would eventually have you jogging two miles a day or doing fifty push-ups or whatever.

Following the pep talk comes the exercise program: "twelve easy steps to health" or "ten simple exercises to make a new you" or "ten minutes a day to win health and fame," et cetera. These programs somehow manage to convey the idea that it is simple and easy. Usually you will get diagrams of skinny men and women bending or stretching or tumbling in ways designed to "take inches off." One author stresses isometrics (about which more later), another aerobics (we'll discuss that, too) or the Canadian exercises or sports like tennis, badminton, and squash. Jogging came into vogue and when that brought a host of sprained tendons and tender heels, the fashion switched to cycling.

Yet throughout all this, the question nags: How do you maintain motivation to exercise? How do you make exercise a habit—a pleasurable habit? Most authorities offer only the pep talk, a program of exercises day by day, and an admonition to make it a habit. The few suggestions that have some foundation in behavior-control science are unwitting and unsystematic.

The real secret of exercise is to habitualize it, to make it as automatic as eating lunch. I will analyze the problem for you and then tell you how I habitualized my own exercise. Unfortunately, since nobody has studied behavior control in exercise (a study urgently needed), I can give you no figures that predict your chances of success. Nor are there any specific tests of any of the behavior-control techniques I will be talking about. However, since such "tricks" work in other areas and since millions of Americans have made exercise into a habit, willy-nilly, you should be able to habitualize exercise more quickly and more lastingly with sound scientific principles than without them.

The Pep Talk

Before we get into the exercise-habit program, I, too, must give you a pep talk. Unless you understand the cost of a sedentary life, you really have no reason to expend the effort and time to exercise. It is easy to fall prey to slogans such as: "When I get the feeling that I want to exercise, I lie down until the feeling goes away." Clever . . . and very discouraging, perhaps deadly. Actually, you pay three major prices for the comfort of doing nothing more than turning the dials on your television or the pages of this book.

First and foremost, your heart. Scientists have accumulated extensive evidence that heart attacks kill sedentary people more readily than physically active men and women. In general, those who do heavy work suffer coronary heart disease at a 25 per cent lower rate (at most) than those who do light work or are sedentary.

In the late 1950's, scientists measured the amount of physical labor among men thirty-five years of age and over in a six-county area of North Dakota. The highest rate of coronary heart disease was among men who did no physical labor at all. The men who spent an hour a day working with their bodies had only a sixth of the coronary-disease rate of the sitters. Each additional hour of hard work reduced the risk until the sixth hour, when it reached its lowest point. At the seventh hour the risk jumped up. At the eighth hour, another increase. However, the men who worked that hard still were in only half the danger of the desk admirals. There are no comparable studies for women, but if all the other scientific data is any guide, the principles apply to women, but five years later.

The Dakota study is important, because it indicates that as far as exercise is concerned, good enough may equal excellent. We will come back to this point again. For the present, it is enough to recognize that an hour of physical labor each day probably produces protection against heart attacks. If you set out to exercise in a regular way, there is some evidence that even ten to twenty minutes a day will afford considerable protection.

Honesty compels me to say that the role of exercise in protecting you against heart attack is doubted by some scientists. Their doubts are based on the absence of any test in which men or women were assigned to groups of exercisers and nonexercisers and then compared. They say that the "natural" experiments in which men who did physical labor were compared with men who were sedentary are flawed because the latter may already have been sick and so selected sedentary work. Regardless of these doubts, the bulk of the data tends to make it safe to say that for the sake of your heart, it is better to be physically active than to sit.

In general, exercise increases the efficiency of the heart, making it beat at a slower rate and push more blood with less work. According to one study, heavy exercise drives down the cholesterol level in your blood. Other evidence suggests that moderate exercise—twenty minutes a day—lowers your blood pressure. There is some indication that exercise promotes the growth of the extra, helping arteries that support a partially clogged coronary artery. However, exercise also makes your blood somewhat more clottable. In an untrained person that is a drawback; heavy exercise could generate a blood clot in the coronary artery. However, a trained individual's blood doesn't clot so readily; he may be protected against blood clots in the coronary artery.

Exercise may also protect the heart by reducing appetite and by burning up extra calories, which will keep weight down. Even though the amount of calories burned up by exercise may be relatively small, if the exercise is sustained on a daily basis and the food intake is kept constant, consistent weight loss is possible. Studies show that youngsters who are overweight eat very little more than those who are not. It is just that the chubby kids simply do not move around much. Even during school exercise periods, overweight children stand around more than their thin classmates.

The appetite may be reduced by exercise. Investigation of completely sedentary adults shows that they eat more than mildly active ones. When adults increase their activity, they also eat more to make up for the extra calories burned—but they do not overeat. The biology of the interaction of exercise and appetite is not well understood. Suffice it to say that if you move more you eat less than if you do not move at all. There is something about the lack of exercise that makes a person eat more food than he needs for energy. The excess is stored as fat. However, if you exercise vigorously, you burn up more calories, and to make up for them you eat more. So, although your appetite increases with more exercise, your food intake does not usually outrun your energy needs and you do not gain weight. Therefore, if you are going to lose weight, exercise may be a critical adjunct to your behavior-control program in that it lessens the power of appetite.

Some medical studies indicate that people who have had a heart attack or who suffer from angina may delay a second attack and reduce the pain of angina through graduated programs of exercise. This is a controversial concept; some physicians claim spectacular results, and others warn that exercise itself can produce a second attack. Obviously, if you are a coronary patient who tries to start out jogging two miles a morning, you are asking for it. Most exercise programs for such patients start out with short, slow walks and progress to longer and longer walks over a period of months. Part of the idea is to encourage the growth of the small, helping arteries of the heart.

If you have had a heart attack or suffer from angina, you might mention these concepts to your doctor. He should know about the scientific studies behind them and advise you accordingly. *But under no circumstances should you start an exercise program on your own if you have had an attack.*

A second price you pay for the sedentary life is that you look like Humpty Dumpty. Stand before a mirror. If you don't exercise, you will see a person with a bulging, saggy belly (no cheating—don't pull your gut in), slightly rounded shoulders, and an awkward stance. Men and women who exercise regularly usually have erect posture, tight, smooth skin, relaxed but firm muscles; they are not flabby or paunchy. Their up, bouncy quality is difficult to pinpoint but it stands out in any group. They look good.

I believe, but I cannot prove, that many of the people who have taken to the jogging tracks, bicycle paths, and tennis courts are more interested in good looks than health. So be it. If vanity prompts people to want to retain their good looks through exercise, rather than through skin painting or grooming, so much the better. And although physical activity—strenuous physical activity—was once reserved almost exclusively for men, women have as much—or more—to gain in the looks department as men. Somehow, society has imposed a stricter standard of beauty on women than on men. The standard is a youthful one. Youth implies vigor, trimness, and firmness: exercise can provide those ingredients much more readily than rouge, lipstick, and permanent waves. Think, for example, of professional dancers who continue to dance long past their fifties. They always seem far younger than their actual years. My wife's first dance instructor, who at this writing is sixty-four, continues to give concert performances, and practices vigorously every day. When she walks along the beach she draws whistles from unsuspecting males who are half her age. She is thin; she walks with much of the sprightliness she had as a young dancer. If you want more recognizable examples, think of Margot Fonteyn, who is past fifty, José Limón, who danced past sixty, and the irrepressible Fred Astaire, who is—what—seventy?

Exercise makes you more conscious of your body, its shape or misshape, and this consciousness can be used to reinforce your thought rewards and punishments in your diet program, providing ready images of a slim, trim you—or the opposite.

The third cost of sitting down in life is the inability to meet emergencies in everyday life. Accidents do happen. You may fall and hurt yourself and be far from help. You may be swept under by a random wave in the ocean. You may be caught in a fire and have to exit quickly or exert some strength to escape. You could be trapped by an automobile breakdown on a lonely road and be without help for hours. Is it far from possibility for you to be on vacation in the mountains and get lost, fall and injure yourself? And finally, there are natural disasters—earthquakes, floods, and the like. Although each of these seems remote, accidents do constitute one of the great threats of modern life. And being in good condition can mean the difference between succumbing to an accident and surviving it.

More Moving Benefits

There is good evidence that if you perform certain kinds of exercises regularly, you can prevent back troubles. And if you already have backaches, exercise may reduce the pain considerably if done frequently and with care.

Regular exercise can improve your sleep, not by making you tired, but by improving your muscle tone, breathing, and heart condition. In fact, any regular physical activity tends to eliminate insomnia. Scientific measurements have shown that exercise also tends to reduce fatigue and irritability. There is common sense in that. If your heart, lungs, and body are trained to work far beyond the daily demands on the job or at home, you certainly won't be put off by low-key daily demands.

All sorts of claims have been made for improved psychological outlook as a result of regular exercise. The evidence is weak at best. I know I feel better mentally when I have been exercising regularly and many others report the same, but that is not proof. It does seem likely, though, that with improved sleep and reduced fatigue and irritability, the general psychological outlook would improve.

Something of the same reasoning goes for sexual activity. It takes physical work to be sexual. If you have little strength or stamina, sex becomes a big physical effort. Despite the rewards of sex, the activity becomes more and more difficult. The habit weakens. There is some suggestion that much of the decrease in sex activity of older persons is due not to reduced sex drive, but to their increasing physical weakness as they become more indolent, gain weight, and lose stamina.

Will regular exercise make you live longer? Scientists argue heatedly over the connection between physical activity and longevity. Some studies of athletes show that they live no longer than anybody else. But that may be because athletes stop exercising as they get older, continue their high-saturated-fat, high-cholesterol diet, gain weight, and become as susceptible as the rest of the population. Furthermore, since good enough equals excellent as far as exercise is concerned, it may be that athletes ·gain little extra by their superb condition. The weight of evidence suggests that exercise does prevent coronary heart attacks; to my mind that means exercise also increases life expectancy.

Good enough equals excellent is one important principle of exercise. This means that there is a minimum amount of physical activity that provides protection and that if you exercise more, you probably gain something but not much. Another principle is: you cannot store up the protective effects of exercise done long ago. If you want protection now, you must be exercising now. Of course, exercising at an early age makes it easier to exercise later at the levels needed to get protection.

What Kind of Exercise?

Before you apply behavior-control methods to make exercise a habit, you should understand the kind of exercise you need and how to keep track of it. It really isn't good enough to run out and start jogging or swimming. You have to know how much and what kind.

The nonathlete need concern himself with only two types of physical fitness: heart-lung fitness—cardiorespiratory fitness (CRF), the most important—and strength and flexibility fitness (S/FF). Athletes also train for timing, skill, and extended stamina, but these need not concern us here.

Besides possibly protecting your heart, CRF helps you lose weight, improves sleep and sex activity, and reduces fatigue. S/FF makes you look and feel good, and sharpens responses in emergencies. Except in cases where isometrics alone are used, the two types of fitness are the interrelated results of an exercise program.

Isometrics—False Fitness

Isometrics can make you strong. Isometric exercises stress your muscles without mobilizing the body. Pushing against a wall, lifting an unliftable object, squeezing your hands together are isometric exercises. Many studies have shown that isometrics increase muscular strength. Football players and wrestlers use isometric programs to increase muscle power.

However, such exercises do little for the heart and lungs. Weightlifters, who come close to being isometricians, have the poorest cardiovascular fitness of any class of athletes. Mr. America may look like a champion piece of beef, but unless he has been running, swimming, or doing something to give his heart and lungs a workout, he is a cardiorespiratory weakling.

Cardiorespiratory Fitness

If you want CRF, you must perform an adequate amount of exercise every week that will give your heart and lungs a workout. How much is adequate? As I mentioned earlier, just one hour of physical labor a day seems to provide protection against coronary heart attacks in middle-aged men. Unfortunately, there is no long-term study of different amounts of self-imposed exercise and heart protection, so one can only make some inspired guesses based on measurements of heart and lungs responding to programs of exercise.

Scientists use two measurements to determine CRF, both of which boil down to the same thing: how efficient your heart-lung system is in delivering oxygen to the rest of your body and how efficiently your body uses that oxygen. Your lungs breathe in air, which is one-fifth oxygen, and your body tissues use the gas to extract energy from chemicals—sugar, fats, protein. Oxygen is what helps you to burn up calories. Heart-lung-tissue efficiency is also known as aerobic efficiency.

Obviously, if you are not in good condition, if your CRF is

low, your body is inefficient. It uses more oxygen and calories to do the same amount of work than another person's does whose CRF is high. Your heart has to work harder to push more blood to feed oxygen to your muscles. Short bursts of work do not measure CRF, because in short bursts the tissues use stored chemicals that release energy without oxygen. It is when tissues must fall back on the oxygen system that CRF becomes important. And that occurs during periods of extended physical activity.

Picture yourself walking up a flight of stairs. You are actually lifting your body nine inches at a time as your legs mount each step. Your heart will beat faster and you will breathe harder as you speed up because you are burning up more calories and need more oxygen to do it. If you are inefficient, your heart will beat very quickly in an effort to get as much oxygen as possible into the tissues. A trained person doing the same work will have a much slower heart rate, because his aerobic capacity is larger.

Ways You Can Measure CRF

Most human beings under the age of thirty-five can race their heart at a maximum of 180 beats a minute; some reach 195. Older persons can get to 160. No matter what the workload, the heart just won't go any faster. At that rate the individual is using as much oxygen as he can. Scientists call it the point of maximum oxygen consumption. The amount of oxygen being used then is a measure of CRF; the more an individual is able to use, the more fit he is and the more work he is able to do at top rates. In the laboratory, scientists capture the individual's breath, measure the pulse rate, and calculate the amount of oxygen being burned as the subject rides a bicycle or walks a treadmill. In this way they make accurate measurements of CRF.

Unfortunately for the man or woman who has not been exercising, such measurements at maximum heart rates are brutal, if not downright dangerous. To get the heart going at 180 beats a minute can be agonizing for the unfit. Not long ago, Kenneth H. Cooper, the ex-Air Force doctor who developed aerobics, an exercise program that stresses cardiorespiratory fitness, invented a measure of maximum oxygen consumption. He called it the twelve-minute walk-run. Its big advantage is that you do not need a laboratory or special instruments, just a clock.

Dr. Cooper's instruction was to run as far as you could in twelve minutes. If you could only run a few minutes, then you walked until you were able to run again. The idea was to go as far as possible in twelve minutes. The distance covered was a measure of the maximum oxygen consumption.

Many cardiac specialists worried about the dangers of such a demanding test for the middle aged. After all, Dr. Cooper had worked it out on healthy Air Force officers and enlisted men. Subsequently, Dr. Cooper warned against taking the twelve-minute test unless you had been exercising at a rather high level for at least six weeks. I agree. Dr. Cooper also invented another test. The subject runs 1.5 miles as fast as he can. The shorter the time, the higher the CRF. Again: if you are over thirty and have not been exercising, do not take the tests. After you are familiar with ways to create an exercise program for yourself, you will know when to take the Cooper test.

The Cooper Fitness Tests

Important: Do not take these tests unless: you have been exercising enough to have reached the intermediate goals (discussed on page 85) for at least three weeks. (Dr. Cooper suggests that you can do the test after exercising six weeks in his program. As you will see, my program is slower than his and my standard is tougher and safer.) All middle-aged men who have been leading sedentary lives should pass a medical test that includes an electrocardiogram with exercise, according to your age. If at any time during the test you feel pain anywhere in your body, STOP.

THE TWELVE-MINUTE RUN. In exercise clothes, walk or run for twelve minutes as far as you can comfortably. If you get winded, slow down and run again when you can. The idea is to go as far as you can in those twelve minutes. When you finish, mark the beginning and end and then measure the distance with your car's odometer; if you ran on a track, count the number of laps. Rate yourself accordingly.

TWELVE-MINUTE TEST* (distance covered in miles)

Age	Very Poor	Poor	Fair	Good	Excellent
Under 30					
Men	<1.00	1.00–1.49	1.25–1.49	1.50–1.74	1.75+
Women	< .95	.95–1.14	1.15–1.34	1.35–1.64	1.65+
30 to 39					
Men	< .95	.95–1.14	1.15–1.39	1.40–1.64	1.65+
Women	< .85	.85–1.04	1.05–1.24	1.25–1.54	1.55+
40 to 49					
Men	< .85	.85–1.04	1.05–1.29	1.30–1.54	1.55+
Women	< .75	.75– .94	.95–1.14	1.15–1.44	1.45+
Over 50					
Men	< .80	.80– .99	1.00–1.24	1.25–1.49	1.50+
Women	< .65	.65– .84	.85–1.04	1.05–1.34	1.35+

< Means less than

THE 1.5-MILE RUN

Measure out a distance of 1.5 miles, either on a track or by driving the distance with your automobile. Then run or walk the distance as fast as you can, slowing down when necessary. If you feel pain, STOP. Check the table for your fitness category. Dr. Cooper did not have enough data for women at the time he published the table; I calculate that for each category and age it should take women about two minutes longer. But that's a rough guess.

Another way of determining your CRF is to take your pulse at rest. Clearly, if you are in good condition and efficiently using oxygen, your heart will work slowly when you are resting. The average resting pulse rate for adults is 72 beats a minute. If your resting pulse is below 70, the chances are that your CRF is high; if it is above 80, your CRF is probably low. Remember, however, resting pulse is only a probable indicator. If you exercise regularly, you will find that in time your resting pulse will go down. If it doesn't, you are probably not exercising enough.

* From *The New Aerobics* by Kenneth H. Cooper (New York: M. Evans, 1970).
© 1970 by Kenneth H. Cooper, M.D. Used with permission.

1.5-MILE TEST* (time in minutes and seconds)

Age	Very Poor	Poor	Fair	Good	Excellent
Under 30	16:30+	16:30–14:31	14:30–12:01	12:00–10:16	<10:15
30 to 39	17:30+	17:30–15:31	15:30–13:01	13:00–11:01	<11:00
40 to 49	18:30+	18:30–16:31	15:30–14:01	14:00–11:31	<11:30
Over 50	19:00+	19:00–17:01	17:00–14:31	14:30–12:31	<12:30

< Means less than

A Submaximal Test

Can you find out if you are in good cardiorespiratory condition without knocking yourself out? Fortunately, scientists have developed tests that do not require maximum effort. They measure your oxygen and heart rates at several different workloads below maximum. Then they calculate what your oxygen consumption should be at 180 heartbeats a minute.

Alas, the tools to measure oxygen and the special bicycles and treadmills that tell precisely how hard you are working are not part of the average household. However, if you have a chair whose seat is eighteen inches off the floor and if you can take your pulse or have somebody take it for you, you can measure your CRF. It will take about ten minutes. You will also have to do some arithmetic. It really isn't necessary to make this measurement *before* you start an exercise program. If you haven't been exercising, your CRF will be low—I can almost guarantee it. However, an actual measurement showing you *how* low may motivate you to start an exercise program. I tested a fellow in my office and he went out and bought a bicycle the next day.

Again, be warned: Don't take the test if you have had heart or lung trouble. Don't take the test if you are 20 per cent or more overweight (see desirable-weight charts, chapter 7). If you are

* From *The New Aerobics* by Kenneth H. Cooper (New York: M. Evans, 1970). © 1970 by Kenneth H. Cooper, M.D. Used with permission.

middle-aged and sedentary, get your heart checked by a doctor. If at any time during the test you feel pain anywhere, STOP.

The chair test depends on the speed with which the heart returns to normal beating after exercise. The higher your CRF score, the faster your heart will return to normal. This correlates roughly with your heart-lung efficiency. From a scientific point of view, the test leaves something to be desired, but it is a good measure for three general categories: poor, average, and excellent. If you fall between average and poor, count it as poor. If you fall between average and excellent count it as average, unless you are closer to excellent, then count it as good. Anything above average is a plus.

STEP ONE: With a watch in your hand step up on the chair once every ten seconds. That will be six times a minute. Continue for two minutes. Measure your pulse for fifteen seconds, multiply by four. Do this immediately after you stop stepping.

If your pulse rate is 100 beats a minute or higher, do not go any further. You are not fit in the cardiorespiratory sense. In fact your fitness is poor. To go on with the next step could be dangerous. If your pulse rate is below 100 beats a minute, go on to the next step.

STEP TWO: Step on and off the chair every two seconds, that is, thirty times a minute, for only *one* minute. If at any time before the minute is up you feel pain, STOP. At the end of that minute wait fifteen seconds and then count your pulse for fifteen seconds; wait fifteen seconds more and count your pulse for fifteen seconds; again wait fifteen seconds and count your pulse fifteen seconds. Then add the three pulse counts for your total score.

Rating	Score
Excellent	61–67
Good	68–89
Average	90–97
Below Average	98–109
Poor	Above 110

The lower the score, the faster your heart has recovered and the lower the heart rate with this exercise. Developed by Dr. Lawrence Golding of Kent State University, this chair test is a variant of the Harvard Step Test, which is somewhat more complicated.

If at any time you feel lightheaded or sore, or get a muscle cramp, STOP. It is no use hurting yourself just to check your CRF.

How to Attain a High CRF

If you want your heart and lungs to be efficient you must exercise them. The accumulating scientific evidence shows clearly that rhythmic, continuous, and demanding physical activity will exercise those organs to the point where you raise your cardiorespiratory fitness. The scientific evidence can be summarized as follows: *To get CRF you must exercise in a way that gets your heart beating at 160 or 150 beats a minute for at least fifteen minutes at least three times a week, or somehow* ACHIEVE THE EQUIVALENT. If you are over forty, you will find 150 difficult to achieve; 140 will do.

Is that hard work? Absolutely. To do something that gets your heart going at 160 for a quarter of an hour is terribly hard. It is near the limit for maximum oxygen intake for most people—180 beats a minute. Obviously you cannot start at that level if you are in poor shape. It is not only dangerous, but painful—and, as we shall see, we want to avoid pain at all costs. Not only that, but as you get older 160 beats a minute becomes more and more difficult to attain. Actually, if you are over forty you may reach only 140 beats a minute. Good enough! So you will have to start out at some level below the maximum for your age and work toward it. The poorer your condition the longer it will take. The older you are the longer it will take.

Of all the programs that have been designed for cardiorespiratory fitness, the best I have seen is Dr. Kenneth Cooper's. He calls it aerobics because it is linked to the efficient use of oxygen. He has written about his work in two books: *Aerobics* and *The New Aerobics*. I recommend the latter because it contains safeguards not included in the first, and it has features for middle-aged men and women. However, because I part company with Dr. Cooper on the psychology of exercise-habit formation, I recommend his book only as a guide to *goals* in exercise.

Dr. Cooper's Programs

Dr. Cooper emphasizes walking, running, cycling, swimming, stationary running, handball, basketball, and squash. All tend to be rhythmic, or at least continuous, and they can be escalated on demand so that you can get your heart ticking rapidly. In the case of handball, basketball, and squash, there is some stop-and-go and a great deal of competition, both of which tend to make many people overstrain. It may be a good idea to hold off plunging into these sports until you have a degree of CRF. (They also have serious drawbacks as habit inducers.)

Dr. Cooper has rated each of these and other exercises according to their capacity to induce cardiorespiratory fitness. He has done it with a clever point system, easy to understand and use. The scheme allows you to achieve the equivalent of 160 beats a minute for fifteen minutes three times a week, without worrying about pulse. It also allows you to work at a lower pulse level for longer periods to achieve the equivalent CRF training. For example, if you walk two miles in thirty minutes you earn the same number of points (2) as running one mile in twelve minutes; or if you run a mile a day in about seven minutes six days a week, you earn the same number of points (30) as running two miles a day three days a week in about fourteen minutes. Dr. Cooper's book provides pages of tables that enable you to design almost any sort of exercise program you want, because they show how much exercise he suggests you do each week to maintain a high CRF level, earning 30 points a week. (These are *goals*, not starting points.)

Dr. Cooper's formulation gives the exerciser the opportunity to control the amount of exercise he does, in the same way that counting calories or following menus provides food-intake control. In case you get to the pool only once a week and running in place bores you, you can develop a program in which you use many different aerobic exercises.

*Maintenance of Cardiorespiratory Fitness**

EXERCISE GOALS

Exercise		Distance Miles	Time (*maximum*) Minutes	Frequency per week
Walking		2.0	24:00–29:00	8
	or	3.0	36:00–43:30	5
	or	4.0	48:00–58:00	4
	or	5.0	60:00–72:30	3
Running		1.0	6:30–7:59	6
	or	1.5	12:00–14:59	5
	or	1.5	9:45–11:59	4
	or	2.0	16:00–19:59	4
	or	2.0	13:00–15:59	3
Cycling		5.0	15:00–19:59	6
	or	6.0	18:00–23:59	5
	or	8.0	24:00–31:59	4
	or	10.0	30:00–39:59	3
		Yards		
Swimming		500	8:20–12:59	8
	or	600	10:00–14:59	6
	or	800	13:20–19:59	5
	or	1000	16:40–24:59	4

* From *The New Aerobics* by Kenneth Cooper (New York: M. Evans, 1970). © 1970 by Kenneth H. Cooper, M.D. Used with permission.

	Duration (*minutes*)	Steps per minute	
Stationary Running	10:00 (morn.) and	70–80	4
	10:00 (eve.)	70–80	5
or			
	15:00	70–80	7
or			
	15:00	80–90	5
or			
	20:00	80–90	5

Exercise Goals for CRF Maintenance

	Duration (*in minutes*)	Action per minutes unless otherwise specified	Frequency per week
Golf	27 holes		7
	or		
	36 holes		5
Handball, basketball, or squash	40		5
	or 50		4
	or 70		3
Rowing	24	20 strokes	7
	or 36	20 strokes	5
	or 54	20 strokes	3
	or 12	30 strokes	7
	or 18	30 strokes	5
Skiing:			
water or snow	40		7
	or 60		5
	or 95		3
cross-country	35		3

	Duration (*in minutes*)	*Action per minutes unless otherwise specified*	*Frequency per week*
Skipping rope	10 (morn.)	70–80 steps	5
	and 10 (eve.)	70–80 steps	5
	or 15	70–80 steps	7
	or 15	80–90 steps	5
	or 20	80–90 steps	4
Stair climbing, ten steps up and down	10	7–8 trips	7
	or 7	10 trips	5
Tennis	20 each	3 sets	7
	or 20 each	4 sets	5
	or 20 each	6 sets	3

These exercise goals were computed from the points ascribed to them by Dr. Cooper. I have included only the exercises that are commonly accessible. Notice that golf is almost useless if done only once a week.

You can interchange the various exercises by using equivalents on different days. For example, if you decide to exercise every day in the week, a weekly calendar might look like this:

Sunday	Skipping rope	15 minutes; 70–80 steps a minute
Monday	Tennis	3 sets, 20 minutes each
Tuesday	Cycling	5 miles in 15–20 minutes
Wednesday	Swimming	600 yards in 10–15 minutes
Thursday	Skiing	40 minutes
Friday	Running	1 mile in 6:30–8 minutes
Saturday	Golf	27 holes (!)

Of course, such a calendar is possible only if you are in good physical condition after you have completed a training period with one or two exercises and do not go to work or behave like a normal human being. In short, for most people such a schedule is a joke. I include it only to show that exercises are interchangeable.

WARNING. Before you begin, make sure you have no physical disability that would make exercise dangerous. If you are under thirty-five and have been to a doctor within the past year and he found nothing wrong with you, it is probably all right to start an exercise program.

If you are over thirty-five, then it is a good idea to consult a doctor and probably have an electrocardiogram taken after exercise to find out if your heart has any problem that precludes vigorous exercise.

If you are more than 20 per cent overweight, you should simultaneously lose weight and start a program that is no more strenuous than walking or light cycling, and not go on to strenuous exercise until you have reached the following intermediate goals and kept to them for *at least three weeks:*

Walking	1.0 mile	in 14 minutes	7 times a week
or			
	2.0 miles	in 30 minutes	7 times a week
Cycling	2.0 miles	in 7 minutes	7 times a week
or			
	4.0 miles	in 15 minutes	7 times a week

If you are over fifty and have not exercised in more than a decade, it is a good idea to start with walking or cycling and reach your intermediate goals before going on to jogging, rope-skipping, swimming, or the more demanding exercises.

These intermediate goals are *goals,* not starting points. You reach them in the same way you are going to reach your final goals—*slowly* and in a way that will build a habit.

Getting Started

Almost all exercise programs—and Dr. Cooper's is no exception—set out a specified number of exercises to do each day or week. You may be instructed to run one mile in 18:30 the first day and continue for a week. Then you are told to increase the effort until at the end of the sixth week you are running the mile in 13:45. Such schedules have two purposes: to improve your cardiovascular fitness substantially, and to do it slowly enough so that you will neither suffer injury nor find it so difficult that you quit.

Although hundreds of thousands of Americans do exercise, every exercise program suffers from a high percentage of dropout, frequently as high as 50 per cent, sometimes higher. We know from fitness population studies that less than 20 per cent of the adult males in America exercise at a level indicated by the goals established by Dr. Cooper; the percentage of women who participate is even lower.

Why don't people stick to the schedules? They are designed for average individuals, which means that close to half the people who go into them will find the amount of exercise uncomfortable. Think of it: you haven't exercised for several years, perhaps never. You are now asked to get into gym clothes and run a mile (to be fair, Dr. Cooper suggests a walking project before running). At its mildest, that effort will set your heart thumping, your chest heaving. You may develop pains in your back, chest, and legs. Every step of the exercise is punishing—and because the behavior is so immediately punishing, it is a powerful deterrent to habit formation. Even if the exercise were not painful, the mere physical effort of doing it works against a habit's being formed.

What to do? The psychological goal—the primary one—of an exercise program is clear: you must reduce punishment and increase reward. The only way to do that is to design an exercise program that fits you, and you alone. Essentially that means increasing the rate of exercise slowly so that at no point do you feel discomfort great enough to overcome the rewards of exercise as you perceive them. That is the key.

What follows does not depart radically from established exercise programs. Your goal is to exercise at a rate that is comfortable and to simultaneously reward yourself for it. (We will come to the rewards later.) Now you want to establish the exercise program that is the least painful. In essence, you want to construct a self-monitoring chart for exercise, and so you must do a few exercise experiments to determine the comfortable rate of increase.

STEP ONE: Pick an exercise that you enjoy, or think you would enjoy. There is a long list of possibilities:

Walking

Running (jogging)

Cycling

Swimming

Rope-skipping (my favorite at the moment)

Rowing

Stationary running

Skiing

All of these are rhythmic, continuous, and easily increased by small fixed amounts (except possibly skiing). Other sports—tennis, fencing, skating, handball, basketball, and squash—have CRF-building potential, but it is difficult to increase slowly the amount you do day by day. You wouldn't think of going skating for only two minutes! It is too much trouble to get to do it in the first place.

Your choice should not only be something you like, but also something that is convenient at the beginning. Walking, running, rope-skipping, and stationary running require no unusual equipment and can be done indoors—a nice convenience in wintertime. If you have an exercise cycle, rowing machine, or treadmill, then you have an even wider choice of convenient exercise. Swimming should be considered as a regular choice only if you are not more than five minutes away from a pool and can get there six months straight. Remember that you can opt for combinations of exercise to make life interesting. The self-monitoring chart becomes a little more complicated, but it may be worth it if it helps you get into the habit.

STEP TWO: Select a time of the day when you are almost certain to be able to exercise. Some people exercise at lunchtime, which has the added value of reducing what you eat. Others do it after work, some before bedtime, some upon arising. I cannot exercise when I wake up. It hurts too much. I do it just before I go to work, after I've been up about two hours. But it should be the same time each day.*

STEP THREE: On the first day, exercise until you feel even the slightest discomfort. You may not even be breathing hard. Okay. That's fine. Stop.

Suppose you select running and run only one block . . . two hundred yards. You feel a little tightness in your chest. Stop. Turn around, walk home. You have found the minimal exercise

---

* Confession: In late 1972, I took a job that precluded exercise before or after work. So I stopped. I'm working on a way to exercise weekends and during worktime. It's tough; at this writing I am having only partial success.

segment (MES). Don't be a hero and try for instant athlete. Don't remember what you did as an eighteen-year-old. Sure, you used to do the mile in 5:30. That was twenty years ago. It is going to take six months to reach the point where you do a mile in . . . what? Ten minutes? The idea is not to do as much as soon as possible, but as little as possible—so that you can build a habit.

No matter what I say, I know that many who read this will try to do much more and go beyond discomfort. Here is how to tell. Five minutes after you stop exercising take your pulse:

If it is still over 100 beats a minute, you exercised too much.

If you feel muscle aches, shin splints, or Charley horses during or after exercise, you did too much.

If you cannot sleep that night, you did too much.

If you felt nausea, lightheadedness, or a burning sensation in your throat, too much.

All wrong, wrong. You should not experience any of these effects if you exercise the correct amount the first day. To make sure you have found the MES, do the same amount the second day at the same time. You should not even be breathing hard. And you should be giving yourself thought rewards (we'll come to these later).

STEP FOUR: On the third day, increase the amount of exercise you are doing a little bit.

For example: Suppose you ran one block and found that to be your MES. On the third day try to increase the distance a little bit and still be comfortable. Perhaps it is a quarter of a block. Fine. That is your daily exercise increment (DEI). You are going to increase the amount of exercise you do every day by that DEI . . . a quarter of a block.

Different people will have different DEI's. In skipping rope, I found that mine was four skips a day; in swimming it is less than a fifth of a lap a day. For you it might be less or more. You will also find that it changes, increasing or decreasing. In my skipping program, I reached two hundred forty skips a day and found that little muscle knots were showing up in my legs. I cut back my DEI to one skip a day for a week, and they disappeared. I was ready to reduce the number of skips even more if those knots in any way became uncomfortable.

On the fourth day, increase your exercise by the same DEI. If it still feels okay, you have found your daily exercise increment and you are ready to make an exercise-monitoring chart.

STEP FIVE: A chart is a simple way of keeping track of your individualized exercise program; you can also use a calendar. Suppose you started on September 1, your MES was one block, and your daily increment (DEI) was, say, an eighth of a block.

Sept. 1 1 block	Sept. 2 1⅛ bl.	Sept. 3 1¼ bl.	Sept. 4 1⅜ bl.	Sept. 5 1½ bl.	Sept. 6 1⅝ bl.	Sept. 7 1¾ bl.
Sept. 8 1⅞ bl.	Sept. 9 2 bl.	Sept. 10 2⅛ bl.	Sept. 11 2¼ bl.	Sept. 12 2⅜ bl.	Sept. 13 2½ bl.	Sept. 14 2⅝ bl.
Sept. 15 2¾ bl.	Sept. 16 2⅞ bl.	Sept. 17 3 bl.	Sept. 18 3⅛ bl.	Sept. 19 3¼ bl.	Sept. 20 3⅜ bl.	Sept. 21 3½ bl.
Sept. 22 3¾ bl.	Sept. 23 3⅞ bl.	Sept. 24 4 bl.	Sept. 25 4⅛ bl.	Sept. 26 4¼ bl.	Sept. 27 4⅜ bl.	Sept. 28 4½ bl.
Sept. 29 4⅝ bl.	Sept. 30 4¾ bl.					

What you have to set for yourself are daily goals based on your daily exercise increment. Do not make a calendar for more than a month at a time. In fact, it may be better to do it a week at a time, in case you want to change your DEI.

To make a chart get yourself a piece of graph paper in any stationery store, or rule your own. Along the bottom mark the dates; up the sides, the amount of exercise, each box equaling your daily exercise increment (see page 90). If your DEI is an eighth of a block in a running program, by the eleventh day you will have *increased* your exercise by ten days times one-eighth, or 1¼ blocks. If you start out running one block each day with a DEI of an eighth of a block, you will run 2¼ blocks on the eleventh day, 2⅜ the twelfth, 2½ the thirteenth, et cetera.

To draw the line of achievement put an x at one block over the first date and put another x at 2¼ blocks over the last date (Sept. 10). Now connect the two x's with a straight line. After you exercise each day, put an x representing the amount you have done over the date. The idea is to stay close to the line.

The exercise chart should be only a guide, not an ironclad rule.

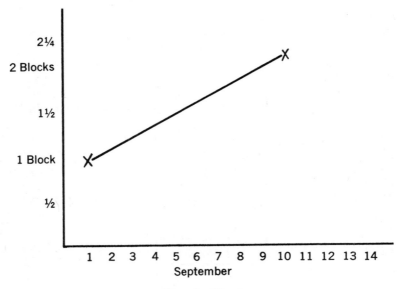

Exercise Chart

Try to increase your exercise as the chart indicates. The following questions and answers might help you get started:

Q. Suppose I want to use more than one kind of exercise?

A. Construct a multiple exercise chart (see page 91). Actually, you can use a single chart for a single exercise if you do that exercise at least three times a week and fill in the other days with other exercises—taking care not to do the others to the point of discomfort. The chart is simply three charts superimposed on one another. On the left, mark off vertically three, or more, different exercises. Then construct each line as if the others were not there, each having its own goal and its own rate of increase. After you do an exercise, use an *x* to indicate the amount you have done. If you do one of the exercises every day, you should have no trouble increasing the amount of, say, skipping, even though you missed five days of it. But if you do have trouble, simply change the incline of that exercise line.

For example, suppose your basic exercise is running and your DEI is an eighth of a block. On Monday, Thursday, and Saturday, you run; on Tuesday, you swim; you cycle on Friday and play tennis on Sunday. Simply follow the chart of your calendar as if you had run on Tuesday, Wednesday, Friday, and Sunday. If your DEI turns out to be too much, reduce it and draw a new chart or calendar.

Above all, make sure that you do not do any of the exercises to the point of discomfort, pain, exhaustion, or lightheadedness.

Q. What happens if I miss a day?

A. Your goal is to exercise every day even if you don't do as much exercise as your chart calls for. If you do something every day, your chances of making exercise a habit are enormously increased. For example, suppose you are at the point where you are running a half mile a day, but on one particular day you have only a few minutes. You should get out and run anyway, even for a few blocks. Put an *x* on your chart indicating how far you have run.

If it is raining, snowing, sleeting, or whatever, making it too uncomfortable to get out and do your regular exercise, have an indoor standby—stationary running, indoor cycle, rowing machine, treadmill, rope-skipping.

But if you do miss a day, go on to the next day as if you had

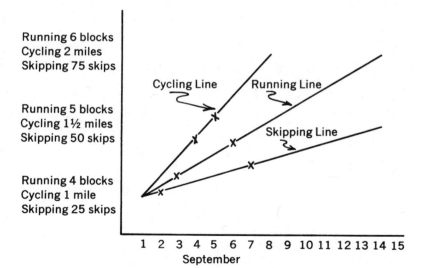

Multiple-Exercise Chart

exercised, unless the increment makes you uncomfortable. If you miss several days, don't try to catch up. Simply shift the chart line (see above) and continue as if you had not missed a thing. If necessary, start at a somewhat lower level. It will simply take you a little longer to reach your long-term goal.

Q. What should I do if I consistently fall below the line, that is, do not make my daily goal?

A. That means your daily exercise increment was too large. Reduce it. You don't get bad marks, but if you try to make your daily goal and it hurts, you won't form a habit—and that is a sin. If you reduce your DEI, redraw your chart (see page 93). You will notice that the achievement line is shallower. If you use a calendar, re-mark it to take into account your reduced DEI. Sometimes you may want to stay on a plateau for a few days while your body gets used to a certain level of exercise. Fine. So long as you resume your increases in no less than a week.

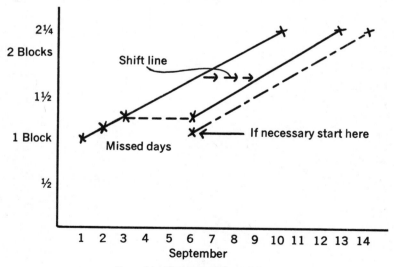

Exercise Chart for Missed Days

What to do if you miss some days: simply shift your achievement line parallel to your original line. If necessary start at a lower level if you feel some discomfort. All it means is that it will take you longer to reach your goal.

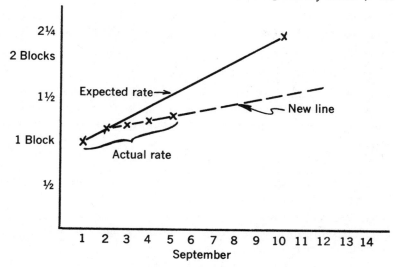

Exercise Chart for Reducing DEI

What to do if you are not keeping up: draw a new line through your actual exercise rates and follow that.

Q. What happens at the end of ten or thirty days?

A. Draw a new chart or fill in a new calendar, using the same or a new DEI to suit your feelings.

Q. How long do I keep this up?

A. The goal is to achieve cardiorespiratory fitness. Dr. Cooper has done extensive work on the various exercises and how much you have to do to get a high CRF. According to his formulation, if you exercise only three times a week, you exercise at a higher level; I prefer a lower level every day. It is better for the habit. You may wish to look at Dr. Cooper's book and make your own long-term goal, using his point system.

Q. About how long will it be before I attain a sufficiently high cardiorespiratory-fitness score?

A. There is no hard and fast rule. It depends on your present physical condition, your age, and, most important, how well you organize your habit-forming rewards. Like crash dieters, many people who want to be in good physical condition get out on the track and run themselves to exhaustion day after day. They will get a high CRF score in a few months, but the chances of their maintaining the habit are about as good as the chances of the crash dieter staying slim. Some do it; most do not.

If you join a physical-fitness program at a Y, gym, or other organization, you will find yourself progressing faster than you would by yourself. However, under the whip of an exercise leader you do not form the self-discipline to hold on to the habit, even though, in a sense, it is easier to get going with somebody calling the beat.

Dr. Cooper lays out a sixteen-week conditioning program. Other scientists have found that three months of high-level exercise is necessary to reduce pulse rate and to increase the CRF score.

Q. When can I play tennis, handball, and other sports?

A. The problem with sports is that they make it difficult to measure exactly the amount of effort involved. There is a lot of stopping time, which doesn't count. Furthermore, there is a tendency in competitive sports to do more than is comfortable. You end up with muscle aches and pains, a condition not conducive to habit formation.

My suggestion is that you do not undertake competitive sports until you are doing at least one of the following daily: ten minutes, at a good rate, of running, stationary running, rope-skipping, cycling, or swimming. For young people the cycling should be done so that you cover at least three miles in those ten minutes; walking should reach a level of 1½ miles in twenty-one minutes; swimming should be at least three hundred yards in seven minutes every day. Older people can have lower goals. In short, you should be close to your final goal before getting into a sport.

A colleague of mine was so imbued with the idea of the need for exercise that he went out and bought a new bicycle. The first day he was out in New York's Central Park for four hours. Three days later he stepped off a curb and pulled a knee tendon. The two events are not unrelated. He overdid the cycling the first day and irritated and weakened that tendon. The first misstep set him up for the damage. You *must* go slowly, not only for habit formation but for safety.

There are many men who believe that getting into a sport and working hard until your tongue hangs out is an expression of manliness. Perhaps. But the fact is that the vast majority of American males do not do any exercise, and even athletes who were in top physical condition when they played fall away. The manly image for exercise, I believe, has also deterred women from undertaking exercise. Now, however, more and more women are taking up dance, both ballet and modern, tennis, skiing, and a few other activities that bid fair to improve their CRF's.

Reward Images

It is an axiom of behavior-control psychology that reward is essential to habit formation. With exercise, the problem is to increase the power of the short-term-reward mechanism over the short-term-punishment. Unfortunately for our purposes, most of the rewards of exercise are long term: possible good health, good looks, good feeling; most of the punishments are immediate: effort, pain, discomfort, and boredom. The exercise enthusiasts say that if you can just get into condition, you will enjoy the jogging, cycling, and swimming. That may be true for some people, but as Dr. Cooper admits, his wife, who jogs alongside him, doesn't like exercise. She does it because she thinks of how nice she will look in a slim dress! Thought reward!

As you exercise you must keep some rewarding thought in mind. Use it to keep going over the effort you are expending. If you feel pain, stop. Of course, athletes use powerful thought rewards and punishments to keep going in spite of extreme pain. When I was on the track squad at college, I ran until my sides ached because I did not want to be last. My teammates ran because the image of winning was very strong. All coaches know that they must somehow instill that image of winning in their teams if they expect them to push through maximal effort, over pain, nausea, and burning sensations. Perhaps that is why athletes quit exercising after they leave competition: the image of winning has gone and there is nothing to replace it. For ordinary people, the thought reward need only be strong enough to carry through the effort.

GOOD LOOKS. This is a good image. As you exercise you see yourself thin, muscular (if you are a man) or svelte (if you are a woman). Try to keep the image going if the effort seems to be verging on the side of discomfort. Again, if you feel pain or any adverse effects, stop. Don't try to override it with the image. Use the image as a reward for your work, not for pain.

It has been my observation that joggers, swimmers, and exercisers in general are somewhat vain about their bodies (I am). If that makes you exercise, okay.

GOOD HEALTH. If you can conjure up an image of yourself in good health, perhaps even visualizing your robust heart beating, you can use it to spur yourself on. Older people, who have intimations of mortality, may find it as powerful as the image of good looks is to younger people.

Since good physical condition also improves sexual ability, you might try using sexual images to spur your exercise program. Indeed, such images may be among the most powerful. Many a middle-aged man starts exercising at the beginning of a love affair.

GOOD FEELING. You will feel better as you exercise—more alert, less achy, less depressed. You can use such an image of yourself to overcome the punishment of effort.

Overcoming Inertia

"Once I get to a gym, I have no problem." A common quote from a would-be exerciser. "I don't like getting dressed and undressed." Another one. Both express the inertia most people have before starting exercise. In behavioral terms, it means that starting the sequence of behavior that leads to exercise is less appetitive than whatever you happen to be doing at the moment. Most exercise programs tell you to exert "willpower." Some tell you to think about how happy you are going to be, which is a form of thought reward. But to overcome inertia, you have to set up a specific behavior-control program.

Exercise at the same time every day. When you do that, the clock becomes a signal (a stimulus) for the start of exercise. Sometimes when I'm deep in some project and I happen to glance up at the clock and it says 9:10 A.M. (my exercise time is 9:00 A.M.), I get a slight feeling of panic and move quickly to start.

Another way of overcoming inertia is to use thought punishments. Typical images: you having a heart attack; you as a big piece of ungainly blubber; you being rejected by someone you care about. Here is the sequence:

• The time comes for exercise and you feel like doing something else.

• Invoke the punishment image.

• It should immediately start you on the first step toward exercise —a movement, taking off your shoes, getting your bicycle.

• The moment you make that movement, invoke the reward thoughts.

If it doesn't work, the punishment image isn't powerful enough. If you cannot find one, it means that you really don't believe that there is a connection between lack of exercise and death, bad looks, bad feeling. I guess you will just have to take your chances that I'm wrong.

Capsule of the Complete Behavior-Control Program

Reread the pep talk in the first part of this chapter. This will help with general motivation, get you to believe exercise is connected to health, good looks, good psyche.

Check for safety. If you are sedentary and middle-aged, have a doctor check the effect of exercise on your heart. If you are more than 15 per cent overweight, do not exercise strenuously until your weight comes down.

Design your own exercise program. Select the exercise you are going to continue for life. Determine the minimal amount without pain. Determine the daily increment. Fill out a calendar or chart. Set your final goals.

Reward images. Use rewarding thoughts to overcome the punishment of exercise effort, not of pain.

Punishment images. Use punishment thoughts to overcome inertia, to get started.

Time. Exercise at the same time every day; it provides a stimulus for exercise.

Some More Helpful Hints

As with diet, it helps to exercise with someone else . . . your spouse, a friend. Gregarious exercise overcomes inertia, provides rewards for continuing through effort punishment. However, a large group is a drawback in that the standard of effort may be too high and induce more pain than can be overcome by the reward of having company. So it is a good idea to find two or three people who are following the same behavior-control program and who understand why one person must stop before another.

Games are more interesting than solitary exercise; it will help if you get interested in a game like tennis. Even though you play only once a week, you can use the thought of playing a better game as a reward for pushing through effort in your jogging, walking, cycling, or whatever. However, as I mentioned earlier, games have a drawback as a basic day-to-day exercise because they are hard to measure, tend to push you beyond discomfort to pain.

Using a point system may help motivate you. Reward yourself with points every time you achieve a psychological goal, that is, start exercising, continue through effort, invoke an image to control behavior, stop when you feel pain, et cetera. Each item gets so many points; you lose points if you fail to achieve the goal. You can set yourself a goal of trying to win a minimum number of psychological points by the end of a week, at which time someone may "pay" you—or you "pay" them. While such techniques may seem childish, let me assure you that they work. If you want to habitualize exercise and believe you may have trouble, I recommend the point system, which is more fully described in chapter 6.

Indoors and Outdoors

If you select an exercise you can do in your own home, the chances of your doing it are much increased because you can do it regardless of the weather. When I travel I take my skip rope along and try to stay at hotels that have swimming pools (I am amazed to find that usually I am the only one in the pool).

The exercises that you can do in your home are stationary running, rope-skipping, machine-cycling, treadmill walking and running, and machine-rowing. I have one friend who has an indoor pool. Those who have large enough basements can set up an indoor track for jogging. Stair-climbing is another possibility.

Indoor exercise tends to be less interesting, of course, than outdoor. For example, one eventual goal in stationary running is to run in place fifteen minutes a day, seven times a week. I'm afraid that many people will find that somewhat boring. I find rope-skipping more interesting because I can change the way I do it: sometimes I jump with one leg, sometimes with two, sometimes alternating. Because it requires skill, it keeps me more alert. A friend of mine has set up a reading stand on his indoor cycle so that he can read while cycling. Having the radio on can also help. Changing exercises from day to day keeps interest high.

Equipment

If you have chosen running, get good running shoes and, if necessary, winter running clothes so that you can continue the exercise year round. Don't run in some old sneakers; you are asking for pain. You can also use the shoes for skipping and stationary running.

Indoor exercise cycles can be purchased for seventy dollars—or ten thousand. The latter comes with all sorts of heart- and oxygen-measuring equipment. However, an indoor exercise cycle should have as minimum equipment a speedometer and a device that will increase effort. Forget about the motorized bicycles that do all the work.

Adjust the tension on the indoor cycle to the point where the effort is comfortable and try to keep the speedometer at 15 m.p.h. (warming up at slow speed at first, and cooling off at slow speed at the end). You then determine your minimum exercise segment and your daily exercise increment and proceed as if you were on an outdoor cycle. During the first several weeks your heart rate will be 110 beats a minute. Eventually, you should be expending an effort that gets your heart beating between 140 and 160 beats a minute. To find out how much to increase the tension, take your pulse when you stop pedaling. Remember, you don't want to start your heart at that rate right away. Approach it slowly, without discomfort.

A treadmill can be had for between two hundred and five thousand dollars, depending on what comes with it. At the least you need a speedometer. It helps, too, if you can regulate the incline of the treadmill: you can eventually decrease the time of exercise by working harder as you walk "uphill." Simply follow your schedule of outdoor walking or jogging.

Rowing machines also provide a workout, if they have tension devices that demand effort from your arms and legs. Some machines are arm movers only. No good. You should be able to move your legs, which means that the seat should slide back and forth. Keep track of the number of strokes, taking care to keep the effort below pain. When your heart is beating between 140 and 160 beats a minute for at least fifteen minutes a day, you have reached your rowing goal (slower rates for older people).

A flight of stairs is a good piece of exercise equipment. The effort of walking up and down is harder than running in place; if you choose to run the stairs, the effort is harder than jogging. The advantage is that it can be done indoors and, because it asks more effort, takes less time. In order for this exercise to do any good, you have to do it for at least ten minutes a day, making between seven and eight round trips a minute up ten steps. That is an eventual goal. In the beginning, walk as many steps as you can with comfort and determine how many more steps per day you want to take (your DEI). If you have pain, stop.

Another piece of equipment, which I don't really recommend, is a punching bag, provided you know how to do it rhythmically. Sorry I can't give you any specifics here. The best I can say is to use the 140-160 heart rate for fifteen minutes a day as an eventual goal. That's an awful lot of punching. There are also teeterboards; well, if they get your heart going, okay.

Forget about springs, weights, shock devices, leather belts, vibrators, massagers, jigglers, and rollers. They are worthless for CRF. They may feel good but they aren't doing a thing for your heart and lungs.

Calisthenics and Such

Now we come to the second kind of fitness: strength and flexibility (S/FF). Of all the rhythmic exercises, swimming provides more S/FF than, say, rope-skipping, because it involves a greater number of different muscles. However, if you want to achieve S/FF that will be helpful in emergencies, provide protection against backaches, and give you taut abdominal muscles, then you need other movements. In calisthenic or dance classes directed by an instructor who keeps the pace at a high level, you may achieve some cardiorespiratory training along with the S/FF. But as for doing fast-paced calisthenics at home alone, the odds are against it. You must do the jogging, running, walking, et cetera.

There are dozens of calisthenic programs designed to make various parts of your body flexible and strong. Almost all work in the same way and the number of combinations and permutations is endless. Beware of any program that promises to be THE program to slim you down or give you "new life." In general, almost any bending and stretching set of exercises will do.

There are two calisthenic programs that have been carefully studied. One, developed by Dr. Thomas Cureton of the University of Illinois, has been adopted by many YMCA's and YWCA's as part of their sports-fitness programs. The other, devised by Dr. Hans Kraus of New York University with Dr. Ruth Weber, is used by some physicians in treating individuals who have back pain. Both men have developed tests that tell you your S/FF score. I think one group of tests is sufficient for our purposes here. I've picked Dr. Kraus's, from his book *Backache, Stress and Tension.*

The Kraus-Weber Tests

The majority of Americans, because they lack minimum S/FF, would fail the Kraus-Weber tests.* Try taking them; but if you

* The drawings that appear here are from *Backache, Stress and Tension* by Hans Kraus (New York: Simon & Schuster, 1965), and are used with permission.

cannot do them easily, you do not have the minimum S/FF—and you are a high risk for muscle and bone problems. At no time during the tests should you feel any pain—if you do, STOP. You have failed that test; you have found out what you want to know, namely, that you have a weakness. If you suffer from back pain, do not do any of the tests; see your doctor.

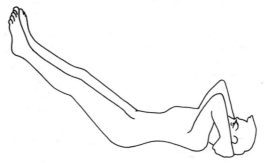

First Test: Lie down on your back with your hands behind your neck. Keep your legs extended, heels touching the floor. Keeping your knees locked and straight, lift your feet ten inches off the floor and hold the position for ten seconds.

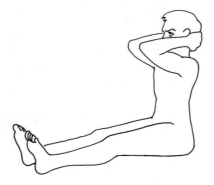

Second Test: Same starting position as in the first test, but this time have somebody hold your feet down by the ankles or lock your toes under a chair or bureau. Keep your hands behind your neck and come up to a sitting position.

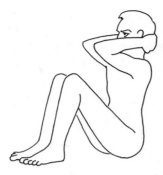

Third Test: This time, on your back as in the first and second tests, bend your knees with your soles flat on the floor. Have somebody hold your ankles or lock them under a chair or other piece of furniture. Keep your hands behind your neck and come up to a sitting position.

Fourth Test: Lie on your stomach with a pillow under your abdomen. Put your hands behind your neck. Have somebody hold your feet and hips down, or lock your feet under a piece of furniture. Raise your trunk off the floor and hold that position for ten seconds.

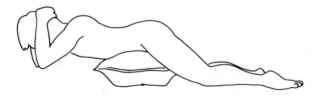

Fifth Test: Same starting position as in the fourth test. This time have somebody hold your hips and back down so that they do not move. Lift your legs and hold that position for ten seconds.

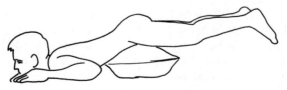

Sixth Test: Now stand up, feet bare, hands at your sides. Keep your feet together and lock your knees straight. Bend at the waist slowly to see how close you can come to touching the floor. Do not bounce or strain. The idea is to touch the floor easily.

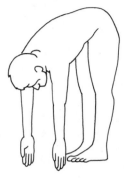

Failure to carry out any of the tests as instructed indicates either a muscle weakness or joint stiffness, which means high risk for future back or neck pain. To improve the situation, you should carry out a program of calisthenics. One way to do it is to convert the Kraus-Weber tests to exercise. If you fail more than four tests you will find the converted K-W exercise very difficult. If you have had backache these exercises might cause pain. So you should probably start with easier exercises, such as Dr. Kraus suggests in his book, or get someone to help you lift your legs or body until you get some strength.

Obviously, if you fail the first K-W test, you cannot start exercising with it. Suppose you cannot even lift both legs. Then try lifting one leg at a time. If you cannot do that, have somebody help you by lifting it; then try to lower it slowly. Try bending your knees and bringing them to your chest. Actually, if you are doing your cardiorespiratory-fitness exercises you will find it easier to do these exercises.

In the second test, try first to sit up in any way you can make it comfortably, without straining. If you cannot sit up with your hands behind your head, try it with your hands extended in front of you. If you cannot do that easily, get into a sitting position and, using your hands to brace yourself on the floor, try lowering your back slowly.

When you find a way to sit up or lie down, repeat it a few times until you feel discomfort. Stop. Do more each day, determining your daily exercise increment in the same way as you did for your cardiorespiratory exercises. About once a week, try to do the next most difficult sitting-up exercise. Do not do it if you feel pain or too much strain. It may take a couple of months, but eventually you will pass the test.

After that, you may want to increase the number of sit-ups you can do week by week. But again, increase slowly. You may find that your daily exercise increment for sit-ups is only one-half— one additional sit-up every two days. It doesn't matter. You will get there eventually.

You may want to go on to sit-ups in which your ankles are not held down. This provides even more training for your back and stomach muscles. Again, if you feel painful strain, don't do it until you have practiced many more sit-ups with your ankles held down.

Do the same with Nos. 3, 4, and 5.

After you pass the Kraus-Weber tests you can introduce more strenuous variations, for example holding No. 1 for more than ten seconds, or opening and closing your legs if you like, or doing a scissors motion with your legs in No. 5, or twisting your trunk in No. 4, or leaning over to touch your elbows to your knees in No. 2, et cetera. Whatever you do, do not push it. Each step should come easily, without pain or discomfort.

Failure on No. 6 indicates a lack of flexibility. You need limbering exercises—stretching to touch the floor in front of you; spreading your legs and touching first one toe and then the other; with hands on hips, rotating your trunk as far as you can to the left and right; sitting on floor with legs straight out in front of you and trying to touch toes with fingertips or to get your head to your knees.

Doing the Kraus-Weber exercises before you do your cardiorespiratory exercises is a good idea. It provides a little warm-up and gets you in the mood for the more demanding CRF exercises. Dr. Kraus suggests that you start each exercise session with breathing in the supine position, emphasizing slow inhaling through the nose and slow exhaling (mouth) while trying to relax.

In all exercises you should make an attempt to breathe deeply and deliberately; slow, deep breathing is better than shallow, rapid breathing. In doing this you will increase your CRF more rapidly.

Continue with your S/FF program for as long as you do your cardiorespiratory exercises—for life. You can make them as strenuous as you want or you can keep them at one level, provided you pass the basic set of tests.

After exercising, it is a good idea to go through the relaxation described in chapter 4. It can be a short relaxation, say five minutes. This will provide a reward after strenuous effort and leave you with a pleasant feeling to which you will want to return; it is also a good time to build up your motivation by practicing rewarding thoughts about exercise. Dr. Krauss contends that stretching and relaxation are the two ingredients that people need most and don't get.

A Recapitulation

Exercise is important. It may protect you against disease. It keeps you looking good by providing a taut, smoothly functioning body. It keeps you feeling good mentally. But to do you any good, exercise must be continued for life. What you did years ago in your youth helps you not at all; in fact, it may be harmful if you were an athlete and then stopped exercising, allowing fat to replace muscle.

Short bursts of exercise in once-a-week tennis, squash, or handball does no good at all, either. And such explosions may be harmful. Ditto attempts to get into condition during a two-week vacation.

Good equals excellent. There is no need to be a superb athlete to get the benefit of exercise.

Use rewards.

Exercise daily.

Avoid pain and punishment.

Slowly. Slowly.

6 / Good Food, Good Health, Good Behavior

You have heard the litany a thousand times: Lose weight . . . Cut down on the fat you eat . . . Eliminate cholesterol . . . Eat a balanced diet. If you are the average American you probably believe some, if not all, of the eating song, but you cannot dance to the tune. Sure, you want to be slim—but only while you are looking in a full-length mirror and tucking in your belly for about ten seconds. You have even tried dieting once or twice. Sometimes you pass up steak because you remember reading something about animal fat. When you order two eggs, easy up, a cholesterol guilt creeps up the back of your neck. Maybe, as an obeisance to the great diet campaign, you will occasionally even eat spinach.

If you have been really serious or desperate about changing your eating habits, you have probably tried some of the fashionable diets: grapefruit and eggs, yogurt and bananas, low-carbohydrate, the Drinking Man's, the Quick Weight Loss, the Air Force, the Mayo, the all-protein, the all-chicken—ad nauseam. If you are a man, you probably started to diet that first summer you couldn't get into your swim trunks. If you are a woman who wears a size nine dress, the drive to be size seven motivates you for weight loss. Yet the diet—any diet—seems to work only for a couple of weeks and then the fat comes flying back to your body as if it were attached by a spring.

Something always goes wrong. A business contact invites you out for a free meal and it is hard to pass up the big steak—when he is paying. Or, after the movies, you always stop off for that big ice-cream sundae. Or there is that terrible weekend at your mother's—eating, eating, eating. Or you sit before the television and, before you know it, you have finished a box of cookies and two Cokes, and you are opening the refrigerator door to get a good-night ham sandwich. Or you cannot seem to control yourself at breakfast (just one more buttered English muffin), lunch (cheeseburger, French fries, and ice cream), coffee break (Danish and . . .), or dinner (three rolls and another helping of beef stew). Each dieter has his own snare. Sometimes it is just the decision, consciously or unconsciously, to enjoy his eating and his weight rather than go on a diet and achieve thinness. Besides, who wants to live forever, anyway?

The Rewards of Eating

The reason for the difficulty is so simple I am amazed that it has not received greater currency in the diet world. All you have to realize is that if reward follows a behavior, the behavior is likely to occur again. If reward follows that behavior repeatedly, a habit forms. Eating is a behavior. The rewards for eating are biological, psychological, and social. They follow eating three or four times a day, year after year (how many meals have you missed?). Only occasionally does punishment follow eating (the food is bad; someone remarks you are overweight). The frequency, manner, choice, and amount of food intake have been thoroughly habitualized by the stimulus-response-reward mechanism of behavior modification. For most people, the mechanism has been unconscious and culturally determined.

The biological reward is clear cut: food supplies the necessary energy to keep the body going. The biological mechanisms of hunger are enormously complex, depending in part on the fullness of the stomach, the sugar levels in the blood, and, it is thought, some kind of internal clock mechanism that tells you when it is time to eat. Hunger pangs (an internal signal) developed through eons of evolution as essential to the obtaining of food and hence species survival. When hunger pangs arise you eat, and those unpleasant feelings promptly subside (a reward for eating). The amount of food you eat on each occasion is governed in part by the amount of food you need to assuage that biological hunger. But that hunger is not the only governor of food intake.

There are also various ways in which eating is a psychological reward. For instance, you may have been taught to eat to reduce the unpleasant feelings of an emotional upset. Jewish mothers traditionally offer food to their offspring when the children have had an emotional trauma. But Jewish mothers are not alone in their prescription of food as medicine for anxiety, which can be defined as a feeling of fear from an unknown origin. Why does food act to meliorate this sense of dread? The onset of anxiety and hunger produce similar body responses: increased heart rate, perspiration, and stomach sensations. If you eat when you are anxious, those biological responses are somewhat reduced. Reward. Eating may not lessen the feelings of anxiety for a long period but it does for the short run, and—such is its rewarding character—that is enough to habitualize an eating response to anxiety. This habit is now a major problem in our society. One side effect of eating is that it makes you sleepy; the drowsiness also softens the discomfort of anxiety. But of course it does not solve the problem of why you are anxious in the first place.

Eating is also a pleasant activity, and most pleasant activities have the effect of countervailing anxiety. Going to the movies, talking to a friend, knitting, playing a game, work (if it is enjoyable)—all quiet anxious feelings. People seem almost to fall into one of two types, according to their response to the many anxiety-provoking situations in our society: one type finds relief in substances—food, drugs, alcohol; the other turns to activities and people. How a person handles anxiety possibly spells the difference between good and bad emotional adjustment, and also—given the bad habits spawned—between life and death.

There is social reward as well. How much you eat and what you eat have been rewarded over the years by the approval of your parents and eating companions. "Eat this squid," an Italian mother may say, "it's good for you." "There's nothing better than a thick steak," says an American businessman to his son. And so it goes, meal after meal. As children we have little choice in what we eat, and after being subjected to an unvarying eating pattern year after year, we learn a "food language" as thoroughly as we do a speaking language. Differing attitudes toward food have shaped the spectacularly different eating styles among Italians, Germans, Japanese, French, and all other ethnic groups.

Even the amount of food you eat is governed in subtle ways by social attitudes. For example, one study indicates that Italian-Americans of all economic classes eat more, and therefore weigh more, than other Americans. With Irish-Americans, only those with low incomes tend to be overweight, as, indeed, are other low-income Americans. The image of gaunt poor is generally an American fiction; the rich are gaunt.

Since you eat at least three times a day, not counting snacks, you have over a thousand eating lessons a year. At each meal, the style and amount of food are reinforced—rewarded—by biological, psychological, and social factors. Multiply that by the number of years you have been eating and you have some idea of the strength of the eating habit. Imagine taking piano lessons three times a day for twenty years, each lesson giving you pleasure. It may not make you into a concert pianist, but I suspect that your fingers would move rather automatically over the keyboard.

Willpower

People often talk about dieting in terms of willpower. "If you exert enough willpower," they say, "you will lose all the weight you want to lose." There seems to be an implicit suggestion that if you fail in this you are somewhat lacking in moral strength. According to the willpower theory, certain foods are "evil"; if you cannot resist evil by willpower, you are a sinner. Thus, thin people cannot understand why overweight people simply don't eat less, since it is just a matter of willpower. So also, nonsmokers do not understand why smokers cannot quit, and teetotalers do not see why it shouldn't be easy to give up drinking.

But scientific evidence suggests that dieting (as well as giving up cigarettes and liquor) has very little to do with willpower in the conventional sense. On the contrary, according to habit-formation theory, a person's style of eating, be he fat or skinny, is mostly a strongly ingrained habit that has been thoroughly reinforced by reward for years and years.

Narrow-Choice Dieting

Most dieters, however, are not interested in knowing a lot of psychological data about themselves. Instead, they seek food information: Is bread fattening? What about carbohydrates, fats, and proteins? They can then narrow their food choices dramatically. They eat only grapefruit and eggs. Or no carbohydrates. Or no bread. Or just chicken. You can see why such diets work: focusing on a simple one-, two-, or three-food menu removes eating stimuli provided by other foods. All the quick-weight-loss diets work in this way. Many dieters have been quite successful in losing weight by thus extinguishing an eating habit. After they lose weight with a fad diet, they try to eat "normally." If they gain weight, they go back to their narrow-choice diet to lose again. If their only concern is esthetics, that is, how they look, such weight-control techniques are fine, but they may not buy much as far as health goes. There is some evidence that seesaw weight loss and weight gain are more deleterious than sustained elevated poundage. Frequent loss and gain within a few months can—some studies suggest—provoke high blood pressure, elevated cholesterol levels, and, in certain individuals, peptic ulcers.

Moreover, such fad diets do little or nothing to change the nutritional content of your diet so that you have the best chance of avoiding a heart attack. Even those diets that are essentially devoid of fat do not help because they cannot be sustained. Low-carbohydrate diets usually mean increased proportions of fat, particularly animal fat, which means elevated cholesterol levels in the blood and increased risk of heart attack. Narrow-choice diets also increase the possibility that you will be depriving yourself of one or another of the nutritionally important foods, producing dietary imbalances and risk of diet-deficiency diseases.

And finally, narrow-choice diets make a significant part of your life boring.

Food Esthetics

Which brings me to the subject of food enjoyment. Many Americans through rationalizing have succeeded in elevating their eating style onto an esthetic plane. They cannot imagine eating a well-done steak. Butter goes with bread. A meal must end with pastry, pie, or ice cream. That is "beautiful eating." Yet it is clear that your taste in food is learned from your parents and from the eaters around you. Italians have one idea of food esthetics, Japanese another, and Americans a third. No one is esthetically superior to the others (although the Japanese is probably the most healthful). It is simply that each group has learned to respond to specific flavor signals.

Cravings

I would not push the analogy too far without more evidence, but it seems to me that foods especially high in sugar or fat have druglike characteristics. A significant number of people exposed to such foods seek them out again, and, deprived of such foods, actually develop a craving for them—behavior similar to that of users of mood-changing drugs. (I would guess that the popularity of French cooking probably rests on the liberal use of butter.) Furthermore, individuals who are used to low-sugar, low-fat foods—like the Japanese—actually experience nausea with the first mouthful of fatty or sweet food, a response observed with alcohol, morphine, heroin, and other addictive drugs.

If You Want to Change Your Eating Habits

If you believe that eating too much or eating the wrong food will shorten your life, then you have the problem of redesigning your eating behavior. There are three requirements: specific, conscious motivation, acquisition of nutritional knowledge, and automatization of a new eating style. I am going to skip, more or less, talking about motivation, discuss nutrition briefly, for now, and concentrate mostly on what I have observed to be the most problematic step in weight loss—new habit formation.

Before plunging into the world of diet-change technique, it is helpful to have in mind a basic store of information about food. There are nutritional assumptions underlying any food-change program:

• To lose weight, the energy content of the food you eat each day must be *less* than the energy you use up each day. Stated another way: you must burn up more calories in your daily living than you eat, producing a calorie deficit. Your body makes up the deficit by burning up stored fat. It is this mobilization of stored fat that causes weight loss.

• To reduce the cholesterol levels in your blood, you must reduce the amount of fat, particularly the amount of animal (saturated) fat, in your diet. Eat less beef, lamb, pork, butter, eggs, ice cream, whole milk, hard or processed cheese, chocolate, coconut, and other foods that contain fats of animal origin. For these you must substitute fish, chicken, turkey, veal, vegetables and vegetable oil, vegetable-oil margarines, cottage cheese, nuts, seeds, and fruit.

• You must make sure that you are getting all the nutrients your body needs. There are many varieties of vegetables, fruits, and fish that will supply the necessary vitamins, proteins, and starches, as well as complement the staple chicken, turkey, and veal.

I have supplied tables farther on, which you can consult for more specific, detailed information. Right now, let's get to the hard part.

Why Don't Diets Work More Often?

The natural variability of human psychology is probably what accounts for the extraordinary number of different diets. All of them depend in some measure on mobilizing the reward/punishment mechanism and on narrowing the choice of food to eliminate the usual eating stimuli. However, most methods too often fail. Why? There are several reasons:

1. The diet pattern is so deeply ingrained that it amounts to an addiction: food provides an emotional reward that fixes the eating behavior as strongly as that of a drug dependency. Dieters often speak of cravings in the same terms as do drug addicts. My suspicion is that anyone 50 per cent overweight falls into this category.

2. There is a severe emotional disturbance in which food is so

substantially rewarding that the individual cannot even bring himself to contemplate dieting; he sees any suggestion of change in his food pattern as particularly threatening. One obese woman, a psychiatrist, told me: "I've tried to diet many times. But when I'm dieting, I get so angry and depressed that I'm mean to my husband and children. I'd rather not be mean, so I don't diet."

3. The new pattern of eating is so alien to the original food habit or so nutritionally lacking that it is impossible to maintain it for any length of time. This is usually true of the narrow-choice diets. The eater gives up and, not knowing a better pattern to use, falls back on his old way of eating.

4. Not enough time is allowed for the change of pattern to take place. To retrain for a new habit is not a short-term project. It takes months—sometimes years—to learn a new way of eating.

5. There is insufficient muscular activity—exercise—during the period in which food changes are made. A sedentary life increases appetite; exercise depresses appetite. Many people feel they eat more after exercise. Perhaps they do, but the net calorie intake beyond what is needed to sustain the body may be less for a person who exercises than for a person who hardly moves at all.

6. The dieter fails to learn to recognize the internal signals of hunger and satiety. Most normal-weight individuals have learned to interpret the feeling of fullness after a meal. Unconsciously, they ask themselves: "Have I eaten enough? Too much?" Obese people have either lost the ability to judge satiety feelings or they never learned it. Neither do they sense hunger in the way non-obese people do. Instead, they depend largely on external signals. The degree of overweight—I believe—is governed by the degree to which you fail to recognize those internal signals.

7. There is a biological impairment caused by the body chemistry converting more of the food intake into fat than is normal. The body seems to need fewer calories to fulfill its energy needs. But this condition is, fortunately, extremely rare. There is also the possibility that the dieter who has always been fat developed extra fat cells at an early age, perhaps as early as two or three years, but certainly before adolescence. When he attempts to lose weight as an adult, the fat content of those cells drops far below normal. It is believed that those fat-deprived cells, by some unknown mechanism, induce hunger.

8. There is a strong circumstantial tide against which it is almost impossible to swim. Often this means a spouse who will not co-operate. In one study of dieting men, the most common reason for not following a prescribed diet was that the wife failed to pitch in and help. Then there are the luncheon companions who make fun of the dieter's attempt to lose weight and who eat highly stimulating foods in his presence (it is not easy to eat a salad when everybody around you has ordered hamburgers), or the mother who insists on feeding the dieter her way and no other. Finally, there is the individual who has inculcated himself only too well with a particular ethnic pattern of food behavior; he feels that the way he has always eaten is the right way.

The reward/punishment technique can overcome almost all of the reasons for failure. The food addict may need some special help from someone—a behavior therapist, perhaps—who can organize the rewards and punishments. When compared experimentally with other weight-loss methods, behavior modification produced the best results.

The person with an emotional problem may need psychological help to bring the problem under control before dieting can begin. However, treatment of the emotional problem does not guarantee that the obese person will lose weight; he will need a method—preferably one involving self-reinforcements—for changing his eating habits.

Similarly, an un-co-operative spouse may be a symptom of some hidden marital disturbance that requires outside counseling. Such a spouse may be using diet opposition as a hostile controlling mechanism. Wives can refuse to cook low-fat foods; husbands can demand steaks, cakes, butter. Once the hidden disturbance is cleared up, the ideal solution for both partners would be to diet together, using the behavior-modification technique. Each dieter can then reinforce the other; each can reward the other.

Reward/Punishment: Slow but Sure

The principle is absolutely simple: you must punish yourself for eating behavior you wish to eliminate; you must reward yourself for eating behavior you wish to habitualize. Simple?

Yes, as a concept, but not easy to do if the idea is completely new to you. I found that once I learned and used the method for cleaning my desk, it was much easier to apply to other habit formation. It may be that you will want to try to form another, simple habit before you tackle dieting.

The first thing you have to understand is that if you are going to lose weight or lower your cholesterol level, you must do it over a relatively long period of time. Remember, you will be working against a lifetime of habit formation; you cannot hope to revise in a few days what has taken years to establish. How long? There is no clear evidence for an optimum time. I think two months is a minimum. If your weight-loss goal is ten pounds, you should lose no more than a pound a week. If it is twenty pounds or more, lose no more than two pounds a week. You will find that in the first week, you will lose more than you planned, because you are losing water from your tissues; also, the early period of any diet is more successful. (Some people can shed five or ten pounds in a week, but it is usually only a temporary triumph.)

While the slow loss of weight has the disadvantage of not providing a high motivation to continue, there are two important advantages: First and most important, losing weight over a period of months gives you time to habitualize the new food pattern, which will not be radically different in calorie intake or food type from your usual eating habits. Second, a reduction of only 500 calories a day means a loss of a pound a week. Such a reduction is relatively easy to accomplish. If you do not count calories, it means eliminating or restricting a few high-calorie foods each day (a pastry, an extra slice of bread at each meal, ice cream). Or, if you have not been exercising, you can engage in exercise every day and not even change the amount of food you eat. But the exercise necessary to use up 500 calories is strenuous and prolonged—say, a half hour of running. If you want to lose twenty pounds or more, you must create a 1,000-calorie daily deficit, which will mean more significant changes in calorie intake.

Aside from losing weight, there is the added problem of changing your food pattern so that you will reduce heart-attack risk. That means switching your concentration from animal to vegetable fats, and introducing the idea of variety. This will require almost as much thought and effort as reducing calories. However, calorie reduction and food changes work hand in hand, because fish, chicken, veal, turkey, vegetables, and fruits have fewer calories than beef, lamb, pork, potatoes, spaghetti, rice, cake, and ice cream. If you try to reduce calorie intake and change food types simultaneously, you will find both easier.

The late Dr. Norman Jolliffe, one of the great nutritionists, theorized that a portion of the brain controls the amount of food consumed. He called that section the "appestat." Like the thermostat that adjusts the heat source in order to keep room temperature constant, the appestat regulates the appetite in order to keep body weight constant in spite of fluctuations in energy expenditure. If a person expends extra energy, he eats more food automatically; if he eats more food than the energy expenditure justifies, the appestat will cause him to eat less food at the next meal. But if, over a long period of time, he deliberately eats more food than the appestat is set for, he will cause this delicate balancing mechanism to reset itself at a higher level. To bring it down again, Dr. Jolliffe suggested less food for a long enough time to allow the biological changes to take place. Physiologists have discovered brain centers that control appetite. If those centers are destroyed in an animal, he will eat almost without stopping. In part, then, it seems likely that in addition to psychological control of food intake there is also a physiological control. But in either case, if you want to bring your weight down you must reduce your calorie intake over a long period of time.

Some doctors suggest amphetamines to reduce appetite. They do work in the short run. Many thousands of persons have lost weight by popping pills. But the loss is usually temporary. Amphetamines also mean a weight loss too rapid for a new eating habit to be established or for the appestat to be reset. The success is far outweighed by the temporary nature of the weight loss and by the possibility of abusing the amphetamines, which are addictive.

Some faddist doctors give injections of mixtures of drugs or provide so-called rainbow pills for weight reduction. These concoctions usually include amphetamines, heart stimulants, and hormones in big doses. They are dangerous to your health while being, at most, temporary weight-loss measures. They are not recommended by most physicians. If you learn to reduce by using pills, then you will find that pills provide the only sure means of losing weight, temporarily.

Should you see a doctor before trying to lose weight? It is up to you. If you lose slowly on a varied diet, nothing untoward can happen to you, provided you stop when you reach optimum weight. If you are 50 per cent or more overweight, there may be something physically wrong with you. It would be wise to find out first.

Because eating is automatic, your eating behavior is governed by signals—stimuli. The sight of food is obviously a signal to start eating. Very few people can look at food and not feel a pang of hunger. A glance at the clock can trigger hunger if the hour is close to your habitual eating time. For others, a television commercial is a signal to get up, wander automatically to the kitchen, and remove something from the refrigerator. There can also be the internal signal of anxiety, to which some people respond as if it were hunger.

True feelings of hunger and satiety are governed internally by a complex interaction of stomach fullness, blood-sugar levels, and certain parts of the brain. Some dieters have reported that after reducing their food intake for a long time, their stomachs have shrunk. Actually, they have learned to recognize a new sense of stomach fullness. There is growing evidence that obese people cannot recognize or interpret the internal signals of hunger and satiety. They eat only in response to external stimuli—sight, odor, and taste of food, the time and location. If they are working in a room with a clock that, unknown to them, has been set ahead to read noon when it is really 11:00 A.M., they will eat if given the opportunity. Non-obese individuals do not react with food drive when the clock is wrong.

Even though a fat person has just eaten a meal, he will eat more if presented with food that looks especially tasty. (If the food tastes awful, the obese person will eat less of it than the non-obese at the same point in the meal.) In a hospital situation, where there is no food around and many of the usual signals are muted or absent, obese people lose weight easily. They respond well to narrow-choice or liquid diets. But when they return to their normal milieu, they resume their habit of responding to external signals that say eat, eat, eat.

Another bit of evidence shows the overweight person's dependence on external signals. In a study of airline pilots who cross many international time zones, those who were overweight felt less discomfort over time-zone changes than those of normal weight. The overweight man simply takes his cues from the clock on the wall, whether it be in London or New York; the normal-weight man is listening to his internal signals and they tell him when he is hungry or sleepy no matter what the clock on the wall says.

It seems probable that if you are 15 per cent overweight, part of your eating habit is controlled by external stimuli—enough to make a difference of a couple of hundred calories a day. And it takes only an extra 200 calories daily—three slices of bread—to end up with an extra fifteen pounds in a year. Therefore, one of the first tasks in any weight-loss or diet-change effort is to recognize the external signals that trigger your eating habit. After you do this, you can take action to change your behavior in two ways:

1. Avoid as many external signals as possible until you fall out of the habit of responding to them. For instance, do not keep high-calorie ready-made food—cookies, pies, cakes, et cetera—in the house. (Narrow-choice diets thus do eliminate stimuli, but it is difficult to stay with them for the time it takes to extinguish habitual food responses.)

2. Learn to stop your eating response in the presence of the signals that are certain to appear. Your new response to the signal of a piece of pie is *not* to eat it. Try to imagine that you are giving yourself a slight electric shock every time you encounter an undesirable food signal. Such signals are, of course, inevitable. For instance, many dieters do quite well during the week, when they pass most of their time at work and away from food. But they lose control on weekends, when abundant food is the natural adjunct of relaxed socializing.

You must also learn to recognize and counter signals that arise in a subtler context. For example, if your previous response to anxiety was identical to that of hunger, you must now be careful to distinguish those conditions and govern your response accordingly.

Before you take action against eating signals, you must identify them. Keeping a detailed daily food diary for two weeks before you start your diet-change project can accomplish this—and you might even start losing weight just by doing it. The sample one-day entry was concocted for a hypothetical obese housewife weighing close to 270 pounds (see pages 122–23). It contains examples of most eating stimuli. As you look it over, you will see that she ate in many different locations, in fact wherever food was available. This is an outrageous example; most overweight people do not respond this way. But I have presented it to show a variety of situations, some of which you will recognize as being frequent in your life.

If you are serious about losing a few pounds permanently, a food diary can be a great help. First of all, knowing the important eating signals in your life means you can deal with them as a matter of conscious will. You will also find out which foods you are hung up on and be able to see what changes you have to make. Remember, too, that variety is an essential ingredient in any healthful diet; the food diary will tell you if your usual diet meets that requirement.

In one successful test of the behavior-therapy method of dieting conducted by Dr. Albert Stunkard at the University of Pennsylvania School of Medicine, the patients objected to the work of keeping such extensive records. But under the prodding of the therapist, they did it for several weeks (which, by the way, shows the importance of getting somebody to help you). One housewife recognized that anger set off her eating. So when she became angry, she avoided the kitchen and wrote down how she felt, thereby decreasing anger and aborting her desire to eat. She successfully restricted the stimulus (anger) by countering it with writing. Each patient agreed that the diary helped him understand his eating pattern. Half the patients lost more than twenty pounds and a third lost more than thirty pounds—and kept them off.

Why do some people start losing weight merely by writing down what they eat? Why do others begin to lose merely by counting calories? Reward/punishment theory provides an answer. Writing down what you eat acts as a deterrent to eating. As you reach for that extra roll you know that you are going to have to write it down, and that knowledge—a punishing thought—is enough to inhibit the act. Counting calories does the same thing: you look at a piece of apple pie—a stimulus to eat. But you know that it is 400 calories. That is a big, punishing number, big enough to stop your taking the pie.

After a while, however, the thought of later having to write down the extra roll seems less and less punishing. And while, if you are counting calories, the high-calorie foods continue to carry sufficient deterrent to eating, the extra helping of moderately rich foods might eventually do you in. An extra slice of bread at *only* 75 calories or a martini (90 calories) seems like no punishment at all.

To change your behavior, therefore, you must figure out and establish a system of stimulus recognition, a punishment for deterring unwanted eating behavior in the presence of the stimulus, and a reward for new, desired behavior. In our lives such rewards and punishments occur by chance or are shaped by our social environment, but we can arrange our own rewards and punishments according to how we want to shape our behavior, particularly the part of our behavior that we want to be automatic and uncontrolled by our will. Further, we can choose behavior that gives us the best chance of a long and healthy life.

The Thought Scheme

The year was 1956. I weighed 190 pounds. For a 5-foot, 10-inch man at the age of thirty, I was thirty-five pounds overweight. I had recently met Dr. Jolliffe, who had asked me with real concern: "Why does a nice guy like you run around looking like a small elephant?" He said he would be glad to help me lose weight. As head of the Nutrition Bureau in the New York City Department of Health, he assigned a nutritionist to set up a new eating pattern for me. Dr. Jolliffe believed that a person's new diet should be close in style to his old one and reduced only in the amount of food. He would not have thought of prescribing a diet for an Italian-American without spaghetti, for instance. Even when he was developing the Prudent Diet, which demands dra-

ONE DAY IN THE FOOD DIARY OF AN OBESE HOUSEWIFE

Start	Finish	Food Type	Amount	Calories	Location	Mood or Stimulus
8:10 A.M.	8:17 A.M.	Orange juice	¾ cup	75	Kitchen	Sleepy
		Ham	2 slices	150		
		Eggs, fried	2	225		
		White toast	2 slices	100		
		Butter	2 pats	75		
			Total:	625		
9:20	9:23	Coffee			Living room	Upset over disarray
		Cookies	3	225		
10:12	10:14	Apple	1	75	Kitchen	Cleaning refrigerator
12:15 P.M.	12:45 P.M.	Pea soup	1 cup	102	Restaurant	Club lunch
		Chicken	½ small	225		Nervous
		French fries	10 small	250		
		String beans	1 portion	20		
		Lettuce salad	1 portion	10		
		Dressing	2 tbs.	220		
		Luncheon rolls	3	180		
		Butter	2 pats	75		
		Ice cream	1 scoop	105		
			Cumulative total:	2112		

		Food	Amount	Calories	Place	Note
3:12	3:40	Coffee Danish pastry	1	220	Neighbor	Elated over lunch
5:30	5:35	Peanuts	8	64	Son's room	Box of peanuts
6:30	7:00	Steak Mashed potatoes Sliced tomatoes Dressing Cola drink Apple pie	7 oz. ½ cup 1 2 tbs. 12 oz. 1 slice	400 150 35 220 150 250	Dining room	To eat with husband
			Cumulative total:	3601		
9:15	9:17	Potato chips	10	80	Watching TV	
11:00	11:10	Ice cream	1 scoop	105	Kitchen	Wanted bed-time snack
			Total for day:	3786		

matic changes in the amount and type of fat eaten, he was careful
not to include suggestions that might be anathema to an average
dieter.

My new diet consisted of about 2,000 calories a day. That was
about 800 calories less than I needed to sustain my corpulence.
Such a calorie deficit meant that I would burn 1.6 pounds of my
own fat every week, or lose about twenty-five pounds in fifteen
weeks. I actually lost twenty pounds in twenty weeks.

Counting calories was easy for me, with my mathematical bent.
At first I carried a little book that gave me the caloric value of
each food. In about two weeks, I had everything memorized.
Before lunch and dinner, I would count the calories I had consumed up to that point in the day and adjust the meal accordingly. Counting before eating is good behavioral therapy:
suppose your daily limit is 2,000 calories and by dinnertime you
have had 1,500. The number symbolizes a punishment because it
will prevent you from having a big dinner. It diverts you—
ideally—from choosing high-calorie foods. Instead of generalized
calorie-counting at the end of the day, counting before eating will
increase the effectiveness of the method.

I had a good diet pattern that was close to my old one; I was
counting calories. Things seemed clear-cut. Intellectually, I knew
exactly what to do. But I loved corned beef, hot dogs, Danish
pastry, ham for breakfast, French-fried potatoes, steak, malted
milks, egg creams (a drink known only in New York, made with
chocolate syrup, milk, and carbonated water; the egg is op-
tional), ice cream, and chocolate bars—all high-calorie, high-fat
foods. Perhaps only dieters will understand when I say that my
taste for these things amounted to craving. I had learned to eat
such foods in a community that valued them highly. I had to
unlearn eating them in large amounts. Dr. Jolliffe urged the use
of willpower to control desire. He used terms such as "cheating"
whenever my weight did not go down as it should. He wanted me
to lose weight over a long period of time so my appestat would be
reset. But my dieting was giving my willpower real trouble.

When my father died of a coronary heart attack eight years
earlier, at the age of forty-four, he, too, was overweight, by nearly
thirty-five pounds. His diet had been extremely rich in fat, just as
mine was. I had become a science reporter in the interim and

wrote regularly on the effects of overeating. I understood only too well the relationship between overweight and my father's misfortune.

In the week just before my father's death, I visited him in the hospital every day, spending long hours with him. I well remember the pale, quivering face. Fear and pain swept over him like angry waves on a dark shore. On the day he died, I arrived a few minutes after his last heartbeat. The intern, thinking he was doing me a favor, drew back the sheet and allowed me to look at my father. The picture of his final agony was burned into my mind: jaw drawn back, mouth slightly open, skin gray; shiny beads of sweat still glistened on his forehead. I shall never forget it.

I recount that sad and terrifying moment for you because of a curious phenomenon that occurred when I began to try to lose weight eight years later: Lunchtime. A cafeteria. The salad counter. The hot table with corned beef, frankfurters, French-fried potatoes. Like an addict, I am drawn to the hot table. I actually hear the rationalization in my mind: Well, it doesn't matter today. I've been *good* so far . . . only 300 calories. I'll make it up at dinner. The stimuli are very strong. At the sight of the corned beef, I can actually feel my jaw working. My habit is very deep indeed. And then an image of my father's face as I last saw it flashes before me. I am appalled. I try to turn off the picture by moving away from the hot table. I take a salad. The picture returns. I shout silently to myself: Stop! I try to think of something pleasant: my forthcoming trip to Europe, a happy afternoon with my little daughter . . . anything to get that hospital scene off the screen of my mind. But note: I ended up with the salad rather than the corned beef. And it happened day after day.

I did not know about behavior therapy until many years later. Indeed, it was not until the experiments with thoughts as reward and punishment were made in the 1960's that I realized the full impact of my experience years before.

The use of thoughts as reward or punishment is enormously convenient if you can make it work, because thoughts are always available. However, each person must find the technique that fits his own life and convenience. Some people find concrete rewards—like money—extraordinarily pertinent and helpful; some cannot conjure up sufficiently rewarding or punishing imaginary scenes; more analytical individuals, like myself, are able to figure out how to pyramid behavioral rewards. It is up to you to select a procedure that suits you and works for you. The important thing is to make it formal, that is, set it up as if it were an operating manual for driving a car.

To begin with, from the point of view of behavior-change theory, let's analyze what happened to me in my attempt to reduce:

1. I am confronted with a stimulus (a signal)—the corned beef at the hot table.

2. The stimulus initiates a response of automatic behavior—I start to reach for the corned beef; my jaw is working.

3. At that moment the unpleasant thought (punishment), the image of my father, appears in my mind. Notice that it occurs *after* the stimulus and simultaneously with the start of the train of behavior but *before* the behavior has been completed. Remember that the longer you wait with punishment, the less effective it is.

4. Instead I take the salad, a desired behavior.

5. Because the image of my father is disturbing, I shut off the thought by shouting, Stop! in my mind. I must do this or else the punishing image will overlap with the desired behavior and perhaps stop that, too. Even if thought-stopping works only for a moment, it is long enough to take the next step.

6. Finally, a pleasant thought as a reward. I used a trip to Europe. I imagined that picture *immediately after* the desired behavior. Rewards work best if they are given after, not before, desired behavior. And the sooner the better.

7. I move rapidly away from the food table. That accomplishes two things: removing the stimulus and providing a high-frequency act—walking. Although you succeed in changing behavior in the presence of a stimulus, the persistence of an old signal in the early stages of behavior change may overwhelm you. So it is always best to get away fast. The high-frequency act, in this case walking, is rewarding in that it reinforces low-frequency acts; the reward is slight but important.

By using thoughts in this way consistently and over a long period, you will instill a new pattern. The method has been used to change behavior in many areas, though it has not been tested systematically in changing diet behavior. But the principles behind it are firmly established; the idea of reward/punishment has been used more successfully than other techniques to reduce overweight individuals. I believe that no matter what method of diet control is used, the reward/punishment idea comes into play at the point of choosing food. If at that moment an individual can think of the bad consequences of his act, he has used a thought punishment. Others call it willpower.

The first concrete step in formalizing your procedure is to make sure you can get your imagination under conscious control. You need to learn three skills: conjuring up an unpleasant thought, stopping that thought, conjuring up a pleasant thought. You have to be able to do all three at will and quickly. After all, you never know when the stimulus for unwanted behavior may present itself. If imagination control doesn't come to you naturally, you have to develop it. Practice this sequence while lying down, relaxed (see chapter on relaxation): 1) high-calorie-food picture in your mind; 2) unpleasant thought (should wipe out food image); 3) stop the thought (should wipe out unpleasant thought); 4) low-calorie-food picture in your mind; 5) pleasant thought (should replace or fuse with low-calorie-food image).

If you leave out the food pictures and simply practice the sequence of unpleasant thought—stop—pleasant thought, you will find that the unpleasant thought loses its potency—in fact, behavior therapists employ this sequence to reduce fear of unpleasant thoughts. Afraid of elevators? A behavior therapist would first get you to lie down and relax. Then he would ask you to imagine yourself in an elevator, then to stop the thought and replace it with a pleasant scene. This would be repeated until the fear of elevators disappeared, that is, until the unpleasant elevator scene becomes innocuous. In light of the effectiveness of this method for eliminating bad thoughts, care must be taken when the bad thought is being used to deter undesired behavior. The power of punishing thoughts can easily be diminished—that is, you will quickly adapt to the thought punishment unless you are careful to make it interrupt the action (taking the corned beef) consistently. You must also make sure that the scene is sufficiently punishing in the first place. The punishing thought also loses power if you do not reward yourself for the desired action.

If you cannot imagine a scene that is sufficiently punishing, perhaps you will discover one in this list:

• Your own death from eating.

• A death scene in which you see yourself as a hugely overweight corpse.

• A picture of yourself as a huge, obese person unable to escape from a sinking ship because you are so fat you cannot fit through the escape hatch.

• Someone you know who is so obese that he disgusts you. Then, as you have often seen it done in the movies, let that person's face dissolve and replace it with your own.

·• A person you love—parent, spouse, or child—rejecting you because of your obesity; think up a detailed scene in which the rejection takes place. (This punishing thought should be used with caution; there is a chance of developing a real resentment toward the person you choose to do the "rejecting.")

• Rolls of fat around your abdomen come off in your hands like sticky, hot taffy—and then grow back instantly.

• A rat eating the hide of a cow or a steak . . . a film dissolve: you are eating it.

The essential feature of such thoughts must be that they are sufficiently horrifying to deter you, even momentarily, from undesirable eating behavior. They must be punishing. If you can stand to think of the scene for a few moments, it is not horrifying enough to work. The rougher its effect, the better will it do its job. Heart-attack victims often have no problem losing weight initially, because they unconsciously use scenes of themselves in the hospital or dead to deter their eating behavior. But in the absence of a system of reward following behavior change, the power of the punishing thoughts eventually diminishes, and the individual begins to feel immortal. The old stimuli regain their power to trigger eating behavior.

In the punishment-stop-reward sequence, the reward must follow immediately after the behavior change. The following scenes are suggestions for thought rewards:

• A beach with the ocean rolling in. You are standing there, thin and beautiful, breathing in the pure air.

• Walking arm in arm with someone you love.

• Playing with children on a smooth, green lawn.

• A thin you standing before a mirror in a bathing suit.

Whatever image you use, it must give you great pleasure; it should almost have the quality of a daydream. Incidentally, sexual fantasies are highly rewarding; they have been used by people to initiate exercise and diet programs.

Getting Down to Work

Now that we have discussed the psychology of eating control and one technique of reward/punishment, you are ready to put them to work in order to lose weight or to change the kind of food you eat (preferably both). In either case, you must act with knowledge and in a conscious systematic way. The emphasis should not be on food but on what you will be doing to change your behavior.

It really makes little difference whether you count calories, restrict or eliminate certain foods, or follow a menu plan. I used to count calories, but now my new pattern is so ingrained that I automatically know how much to eat without thinking about it. Regardless of which plan you choose, try to be consistent. If you are going to count calories, count them every day; if you are going to restrict or eliminate foods, be specific about which ones—draw up a written list if necessary. If your method is to be menus, remember that it takes careful advance planning. Consistency will be easier to maintain as the method becomes a habit.

You must also introduce a variety of foods into your diet for nutrition's sake. Thus single-food diets can be dangerous, even though they work well in helping you reduce by eliminating many food stimuli.

You must end up each day having eaten less food than is required to keep the energy balance in your body. That is the only way to lose. Unfortunately, habit often overrules plan. Calorie counters find themselves wolfing down a piece of apple pie when they "could not resist it any longer." When they count up the calories later in the day, the thought of having "broken the diet" is so punishing that they give up counting. But remember that in the reward/punishment system, there is no such thing as "breaking the diet." Instead, you are concerned with achieving control *at the moment of eating.* Occasional failure even at that point is not important, because behavior can be habitualized even if you sometimes fail to adhere to the reward/punishment scheme. The important thing is to adhere to it *more often than not.* I cannot emphasize this too much. With reward/punishment methods occasional failures are not critical; the idea is to keep the method moving forward by keeping at it systematically.

Yet you must eat less. To keep track of your food intake, I suggest you make a chart for yourself. It is a simple graph developed by Dr. Norman Jolliffe. The vertical scale is marked off in pounds, the horizontal in weeks. An *x* marks weight on the first day, and another *x* is placed at the desired weight after fifteen weeks. On the sample graph shown (see below), the projected weight is twenty pounds in fifteen weeks, or just a little over a pound a week.

On your own graph connect the two *x*'s with a line—that's your weight-loss line. At least twice a week, weigh yourself and put a dot on the chart corresponding to the weight and date. (If you do not have a scale, invest in one. The cost is not a factor when you consider the number of medical bills you will be spared.)

You will notice a rapid weight loss at the beginning, usually caused by water loss. Ideally, loss should slow down, otherwise the new eating habit will not be learned. For some persons rapid

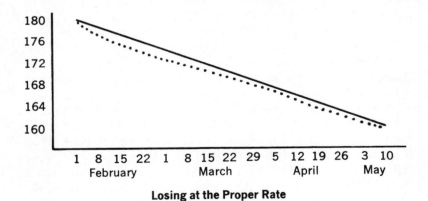

Losing at the Proper Rate

Weigh yourself at least twice a week, at the same time of day, and put a dot on the chart corresponding to your weight and the date. The dotted line shows the proper weight-loss rate.

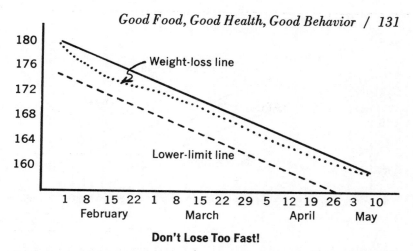

Don't Lose Too Fast!

To keep yourself from losing too fast, make sure your weight-loss dots stay between the lines.

weight loss may also generate peptic ulcers. In order to be able to spot rapid weight loss, draw a second line parallel to and slightly below your projected weight-loss line. Then make sure that the line formed by the dots, showing your actual weight loss, remains between the projected weight-loss line and the second, lower-limit line (see above). If you cross the second line, you are losing weight too fast. Slow down.

The typical fad dieter can lose six pounds in one week, three in the next. Then things slow down and finally there is the inexorable weight regain (see page 132). He never learned a new style of eating.

If you keep your food intake at the proper level, the dots will stay between the two lines. If you eat too much in any week, the dots will touch or cross the top line (see page 133). All you need do then is decrease the amount of food you are eating and the dots will dutifully fall between the two lines again. Your weight loss is strictly controlled by your food intake and the amount of energy you expend. "I've cut down on my eating and I still can't lose" is the typical cry of the dieter and is typically nonsense. Of course, if you have been playing tennis for an hour every day and stop playing when you start dieting, your calorie needs will drop. The food-intake decrease may just equal the number of calories

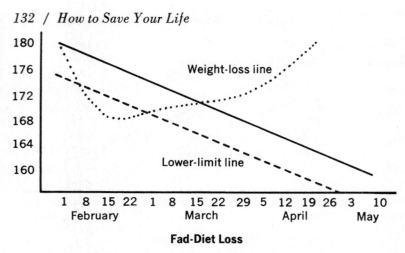

Fad-Diet Loss

The typical fad dieter loses weight rapidly and then regains it because no learning has taken place.

you had used playing tennis. But ordinarily, if you eat less you will lose weight. Your chart will confirm that.

As may have occurred to you, a chart has some reward/punishment features. Crossing a line is a punishment and keeping between the lines is a reward. However, since both reward and punishment come long after the behavior, the chart is only indirectly effective as a behavior-control mechanism. You can increase its power if you use an image of the chart as a punishment to deter eating behavior in the face of a stimulus. For instance, you are about to reach for an extra slice of bread; in your mind you picture the chart with the line representing your weight crossing the projected weight-loss line. That will deter your taking the extra slice if the chart has come to mean something important to you. Even without its psychological utility, the chart is absolutely essential as a method of monitoring the amount of food you eat.

After you have chosen your technique—calories, restriction, or menus—and set up a chart, you still face the major problem of handling eating behavior in the presence of a stimulus. The critical instant, as every dieter knows, is at the moment of the presentation of the eating stimulus. You must control that in order to avoid starting a chain of unhealthy behavior.

Of the two choices open to you—avoiding the stimulus or inhibiting the train of eating behavior when the signal appears— stopping behavior is the more powerful, because every refusal increases your resistance: if you turn down a proffered piece of pie once, your ability to refuse the next time is greater.

Avoiding stimuli, however, is a good strategy for starting behavior modification because it is easier to do. If you have kept a food diary you will have identified most of your important stimuli. What you will then need are some tactics for avoiding them (see pages 134–35). If you find yourself eating in many different places, confine your eating to one room and at one particular seat at the table. If you raid the refrigerator or cookie jar or cake box, simply do not have any high-calorie ready-to-eat food in the house. One mother I know says she has to have such things in the house "for the children." Of course, the children can easily do without cookies, cake, candy, nuts, and the rest.

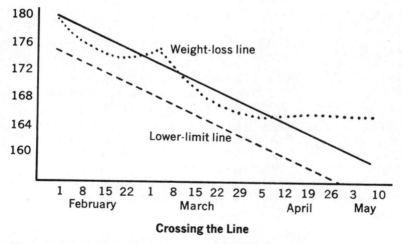

Crossing the Line

Here the attempt at weight loss has faltered, so that the line representing actual weight crosses the projected weight-loss line. A reduction in food intake turns the curve down again. (If the actual-weight line goes too far to the right, it is better to make a new chart and start again rather than attempt to speed up weight loss.)

Far from showing love and concern (or maybe she is trying to buy her children's affection?), the mother is actually injuring them, because such "treats" establish unhealthy eating patterns that the children will find difficult or impossible to change in adulthood.

Tactics for Controlling Eating Response

External eating stimulus	Stimulus avoidance and alternative activities
Multiple eating locations	Confine eating to one location and same place at table. Leave location while the stimulus is still active.
Television	Do not have food near you while watching TV. If a commercial acts as stimulus, leave it on but do not rise for food; talk to spouse or skim a magazine, newspaper, or book. If necessary, turn off TV and leave room; go for a walk or telephone a friend. Do not have high-calorie ready-made food in house.
Reading	Do not have food near you. Change reading location.
Fast eating	Do not put extra helpings of food on the table. Take only one portion. Count mouthfuls; pause on third or fourth. Leave some food on plate or, after you have eaten part of it, throw the rest away.
Anger or other emotion	Leave scene of food. Write down why you are angry. Visit or telephone a friend or relative. Do not have high-calorie ready-made food in house.
Favorite food	Doctor it with a bitter flavor or oversalt it. Do not order, buy, or make this food; create a low-calorie variant.
Coffee wagon at office	Leave area until wagon goes away or order only coffee, tea, or juice. Keep celery or carrot sticks at desk (to be used only as a last resort, when all else fails). Chew sugarless gum (I don't really like this). Make a telephone call.

External eating stimulus	*Stimulus avoidance and alternative activities*
Evening	Talk to spouse, read, or go for a walk. Arrange an outing that will keep you away until it is time to go to bed. Play a game that makes you sleepy. Do not have high-calorie ready-made food in the house.
Bedtime	Talk to spouse, read, or, if possible, call a friend and talk until you get sleepy. Last resort: get some carrot and celery sticks ready, but keep them far from the bed. Once again: do not have high-calorie ready-made food in the house.

Notice that fast eating is a stimulus. Most overweight people eat quickly; in a sense, they do not enjoy the full taste of each mouthful. If you watch them, you will see that while they chew one mouthful, they scoop up a second. Then, as they swallow, they are simultaneously moving the ready forkful to their mouths. The swallowing acts as a stimulus for refilling the mouth. If an internal signal of satiety arises, it is overridden by the signal to continue eating that results from swallowing in the presence of more food on the plate.

To avoid the swallowing stimulus, you must eat slowly. One way is to count every mouthful and pause after you swallow it before taking the next. Or you can lay down your knife and fork after every third or fourth mouthful and pause, perhaps talk to your dinner companion. It sounds childish, I know, but if you do it you will get a sense of control over your eating. You may actually enjoy your food more as the taste lingers in your mouth.

Fast eaters also tend to clean their plates. So take only a serving of food you intend to eat. Better still, leave something uneaten on your plate, perhaps a fourth of what was there. In a restaurant, where you do not control the portion size, leave some food uneaten, even if it outrages your sense of economy. This gives you a way to control behavior in the presence of the stimulus and also reduces your intake. I first heard about this method from a fellow science writer, Robert Goldman, who lost some forty pounds and kept them off. He incorporated the idea in his

book *Lose Weight and Live,* which is full of food-control techniques that work well with behavior modification.

Examine the stimuli I have presented and compare them with
those you have identified in your food diary. Then plot out some
tactics for avoiding them the next time they appear. Each person
must develop his own strategy.

As I said, inhibiting or stopping behavior is more powerful
than avoiding stimuli. The most convenient technique for accomplishing this is thought punishment. To review the sequence once
more: *stimulus,* television commercial, for instance; *food desire,*
actually the start of a train of eating behavior; *punishment
thought,* a fat person—yourself—unable to get off a sinking ship;
behavior is inhibited, you remain seated; *stop the thought; alternative activity,* you pick up a book or a magazine kept near at hand
or talk to your spouse or companion (in a meal situation, another
alternative activity would be to eat a low-calorie food or take a
drink of water): *pleasant thought,* walking along a beach, for instance, held long enough so that the eating stimulus (the commercial) ends.

Each success in stopping behavior makes the next effort easier,
because the power of the stimulus to make you feel hungry will be
reduced—and that will reduce your food intake. An occasional
failure is of no importance, but make sure your successes out-
number your failures.

How well does it work? There have been experiments indicating that reward/punishment methods work best in reducing
overweight individuals. And it worked well for me. After my
initial weight loss some years ago, my weight fluctuated between
163 pounds and 167 pounds. I had always wanted to get to 155
pounds, my optimal weight, but never seemed able to. In the
process of writing this chapter, I decided to give the thought-
punishment idea a conscious trial. At this writing, I weigh 157
pounds.

In a University of Pennsylvania weight-loss experiment conducted by Dr. Albert Stunkard, the patients used points in a
reward/punishment scheme. Each patient set up a system
whereby points would be awarded for each act of avoiding a high-
calorie food situation or for stopping behavior by successfully

countering a recognized eating stimulus. For example, if at dinner a patient were able to put his knife and fork down after every third mouthful, he gave himself ten points; he lost ten points if he were unsuccessful in putting down his eating tools.

Example of the Point System

Behavior Control Act	Points
Left food on plate	5
Paused after each mouthful	3
Invoked thought punishment to refuse high-calorie food	15
Called friend when anxiety occurred	10
Counted calories before meal	5

These behavior-control acts are only samples. Each person must decide for himself what the critical control points are and reward or punish himself accordingly. Remember: you add points for success, subtract for failure. A money pay-off for a positive score at the end of the day will help increase the power of the point system.

Notice that points are lost or gained for specific behavior-control acts, not for weight loss. The weight-loss chart provides the general guide for food intake; the point system has the advantage of immediate punishment for failure to counter a stimulus; point gain is a reward for success.

To make your point system effective, you might get a friend or your spouse to give you money at the end of the day or week for points acquired—and to collect money from you for minus points. It need not be much; a penny a point will do. I have a feeling that a small amount of money works better than a large sum. In general, if you undertake behavior modification with another person you will have an easier time of it and a greater chance of success.

If I were establishing a point system for myself, I would give myself high scores for being able to switch off behavior using a thought as reward or punishment. If you make this skill very strong, you can use it for other habit-forming and habit-breaking needs.

Building New Tastes

It is almost impossible to create a reasonably satisfying weight-loss diet unless you use fish, chicken, cottage cheese, and a variety of vegetables. So a very important part of changing your food style is to learn to like many foods to which you are now indifferent or which you actually hate. It is not enough to merely tolerate the new food; you must actively enjoy it. Suppose you hate fish. Actually, you learned to hate it by chance . . . maybe your mother didn't like it, or the bones frightened you as a child. But there is nothing intrinsically unlikable about fish. Millions of Japanese, French, Italians, and Americans love it. Using reward/punishment methods you can learn to love it, too . . . and it may save your life.

An easy way to start learning to enjoy a new food is to use it in a tasty recipe. There are many low-calorie cookbooks that provide a variety of recipes. My favorite is *Live High on Low Fat* by Sylvia Rosenthal. But at this point, the important thing is to select a recipe you think you will like, even a high-calorie one if necessary.

Silently congratulate yourself (a form of thought reward) on eating the new-tasting food and attempt to savor it. If you have a dieting agreement with your spouse, congratulations can be given out loud; or, by controlling your imagination, you can invoke a pleasant image after each bite. It is a good idea to serve the new food along with something you really like; take a bite of the new food, swallow, and then take a bite of the food you like. If you want to get fancy, you can reward yourself randomly after each bite, or score the eating of this new food with high points. Serve the new food at least twice a week, perhaps three times.

After a few successful meals with the new food, say, veal, you next serve the dish without its high-calorie ingredient—veal with tomato sauce instead of Parmesan. Or you can substitute cottage cheese. Follow the same sequence of self-congratulations, pleasant scenes, serving it with food you enjoy, and high-point scores. After a couple of weeks, you can start trying other low-fat veal dishes. Probably by that time, you will actually like veal and will no longer need to use behavior-control techniques to eat it. It takes from four to eight weeks, depending on how often you serve the new food.

If you dislike a food—say, fish—to the point where you do not think there is any form in which it could pass your mouth, you can still learn to like it. Liking fish is very important, because it is low in calories and low in the kind of fat that has been associated with a high cholesterol level in the blood, which signals increased risk of heart attack. Vegetables trouble many people who simply dote on French-fried potatoes and who would not think of eating string beans, lettuce, spinach, carrots, or any of the items that are essential to creating a varied diet.

How do you overcome hate, disgust, fear? You are by now familiar with the well-established procedure for doing so. It is derived directly from reward/punishment theory and works by desensitizing your emotions at the thought of the item you do not like. The method has reduced fear of elevators, flying, snakes, et cetera—and it can reduce your hatred of fish. It doesn't matter too much how you came to hate it; all that really counts is that the sight of fish creates an aversion to the eating stimulus. You have to turn that around. First make a list of situations in which fish food appears. For example:

• Tuna fish in a can.
• Tuna fish scooped out of the can onto a plate.
• Tuna fish being mixed with mayonnaise (I hope you like mayonnaise).
• You are sitting at a table and the tuna fish is placed in front of you.
• You are eating the tuna fish.

Notice that the list of images increases in the power to make you feel uncomfortable. With this list you are ready to desensitize.

Lie down and relax (see chapter on relaxation). Think of the first image—tuna in a can. If it makes you uncomfortable, stop the thought and switch to a pleasant scene. Wait a minute or two, then think of the tuna can again. The moment you feel uncomfortable, stop the thought and invoke the pleasant image. You will find that the unpleasant image makes you a little less uncomfortable each time, until it is not uncomfortable at all. At that point, go to the next unpleasant image. If this point isn't reached until the second day, start with the first image to be sure that you are comfortable with it. In this way you progress to the last, most distasteful image: you are eating the tuna fish. As you go along, try to visualize the taste and odor of the tuna so that you can manage your feelings when you get to the "worst" image. You can do all this in bed just before going to sleep.

The scheme in outline is: relax—invoke unpleasant thought— stop thought—invoke pleasant thought—relax. Repeat. Notice the difference between this and the scheme for changing unwanted behavior: stimulus—unpleasant thought (stops unwanted behavior)—stop thought—desired behavior—pleasant thought (or alternative activity). The first scheme is designed to make you adapt (desensitize) to an unpleasant thought; the second is designed to deter an unwanted behavior and to retain the power of the unpleasant thought.

After you can visualize yourself actively eating tuna fish without any uncomfortable feelings, you are ready to go on to the real thing. If at the first bite you get a sense of distaste, stop; think of a pleasant scene and try again (or have something on your plate that you really like and take a bite of that). If you do eat some fish, follow with a pleasant scene, self-congratulation, points, and a nibble of some food you enjoy. Repeat until you have eaten enough just to feel comfortable. Repeat several days later.

Of course, it need not be tuna salad. I would suggest some elegant fish recipe that you would have the least trouble eating: filet of sole amandine, broiled brook trout, fried shrimp. Once you have made the breakthrough, you can go on to other fish recipes (using desensitization if necessary), finally eliminating the high-calorie content: the butter, cheese, or whatever.

Once you know how to use desensitization you can learn to like almost any food. (It is also extremely handy in dealing with problems of sleep, sex, and other activities where habits are involved.) If you eat a new food consistently for many months, you will build an entirely new taste structure. If you switch from beef, lamb, pork, pie, cake, butter, cheese, and ice cream to fish, fowl, veal, fruit, and vegetables, you will not only make it easier to lose weight; you will also have a good chance of lowering your blood cholesterol. I know, for example, that after several years of eating very little beef—after having been a big steak-and-potatoes man—I now can eat it in only small amounts; ditto ice cream. On the other hand, as a child I disliked fish intensely. Now I eat it with relish at least seven times a week, often twice a day.

I know that to many of you all of the foregoing sounds too mechanical, as if you would be treating yourself like an animal in a psychology laboratory. But we must all recognize that part of our nature responds animal-like to stimuli and to reward/punishment learning techniques. What makes us human is our ability to use our uniquely human faculties—thinking, sensitivity, intuition, and speech—consciously to control and to modify these animal-like responses. Unlike any other animal, we can arrange the sequence of reward and punishment to suit our needs for behavior modification. Most other animal species' behavior is shaped by reward/punishment systems that are either accidents of environment or biological determinants of survival.

Simple willpower cannot often alter long-established behavior that carries powerful, reinforcing rewards, like eating, smoking, drugs, alcohol, or sex. These behavior patterns have become automatic responses to stimuli that constantly appear before us. Although it may help to understand the origin of emotional problems that make it difficult for an individual to make behavior modifications with conscious reward/punishment, the growing evidence is that a direct attack on behavior, by-passing emotional problems, is often fruitful not only in changing behavior, but in ameliorating emotional disturbances. After all, undesirable behavior is in itself emotionally disturbing.

A good example is provided by an experiment done with patients suffering from anorexia nervosa. The ailment causes the victim to *lose* appetite and weight precipitously: fifty pounds or more in the space of weeks. It is often lethal. Until recently, almost all methods—medical and psychiatric—failed.

Dr. Albert Stunkard, who is professor of psychiatry at the University of Pennsylvania School of Medicine, designed reward/punishment methods for anorexia nervosa patients. Observing the female patients, Dr. Stunkard noted that they were always moving around: walking up and down corridors, getting in and out of bed, and so on. Despite their starved state, they walked almost seven miles a day as revealed by pedometer measurements. (The normal woman walks fewer than five miles a day.)

Dr. Stunkard and his colleagues first decided to restrict the patients' activity; that is, they were confined to their rooms. Then each was told that she could have unlimited activity outside the hospital for six hours on any day when she tipped the scales at least eight ounces above the previous morning's weight. All the patients then began rapid weight gain, averaging five pounds a week for the first three weeks. One patient had lost a third of her weight with the onset of anorexia; she was 90 pounds when she reached the hospital; she gained twenty pounds under the reward regime.

Although the anorexia patients gained weight and stayed alive, they still suffered from severe mental disturbances. This example is only meant to illustrate that behavior therapy can operate even in the presence of emotional problems if you can find rewards and punishments powerful enough.

Individuals with relatively few emotional problems (who is entirely free of them?) will find behavior modification easy to use; they will not be sidetracked by psychological issues. They will find it possible to learn a new style of eating and discover that there is nothing so holy about the flavor of an eight-ounce steak that it must be placed above a delicately broiled filet of sole. They will travel widely in the country of culinary tastes—at the same time decreasing the risk of certain diseases, and feeling as good as they look.

If you believe you can do all this by "willpower" alone, good luck. Some have succeeded; but many more have failed.

7 / Food Facts You Need to Know

In America only a hermit would not know that weight reduction and cholesterol control may be of some health importance. True, there is controversy over these matters, particularly cholesterol. Yet, as we shall see, there is some evidence for believing that taking the cholesterol out of your blood may be more important than weight reduction in extending life. If you have made up your mind to improve your weight and cholesterol situation, it is helpful to understand why you are doing it.

If you have been avoiding reading anything about food and health and have been going to the table like a sleepwalker, you should know that if you eat too much food or the wrong food, you will shorten your life. And a shortened life also means, in general, a sicker life, a less useful one, and, ultimately, a more painful one. By following the high-calorie, high-animal-fat American pattern of eating, you are trading short-term enjoyment for long-term pain. As with any habitual activity, the psychological reward of, say, a thick steak is far more reinforcing of the habit at the moment of eating than is the punishing power of the anticipation of pain and early death some years after the steak is consumed. But if you learn what the bridges are between food and death, and, more important, between food and life, a commitment to a new nutrition will seem worthwhile and thereby easier.

Atherosclerosis

One disease more than any other derives from a food pattern that emphasizes animal fats and high calories. It is also connected to a sedentary life, perhaps to a high-pressure life, and certainly to heredity. It is the biggest killer of all—accounting for half the deaths in the United States—responsible for heart attacks, strokes, and, in part, high blood pressure. It reduces life expectancy in middle-aged men by between eight and twelve years. While not so damaging for middle-aged women, it also cuts life short for them and often batters their brains into insensibility, leaving them vegetables in their later years.

The disease attacks the blood vessels, clogging them with a greasy whitish material. Ultimately, the disease so narrows the vessels that blood flow slows or stops altogether. Scientists call the ailment "atherosclerosis." *Athero,* from the Greek, means "grain." The inner surface of the diseased channel has a grainy appearance from the deposits; it looks something like cooked barley. *Sclerosis,* also from the Greek, means "hardened." The fatty, grainy deposits stiffen the artery. Sometimes the disease is called "arteriosclerosis" because it almost always attacks arteries, the vessels that carry fresh, oxygenated blood from the heart to the rest of the body.

There is a saying that you are as old as your arteries. The more clogged they are, the more infirmities you suffer. If atherosclerosis jams the tubes feeding blood to your brain, you are in line for a stroke. You can readily understand that if the pipes leading to your thinking machine are lined with scale, you have much less blood flowing to the gray matter. The sick arteries' grainy lining also provides good anchor for blood clots and if one should form in a brain artery, the clot shuts off blood flow to a portion of the brain. Since nerve cells die rapidly if deprived of oxygen (carried by blood), portions of the brain die. A nerve cell can survive about four to six minutes without blood. If the shutdown is widespread, whole nerve networks collapse and organ systems all over the body stop functioning; often death, mercifully, intervenes.

But some stroke victims are not lucky enough to die. Only part of the brain dies, so only a few organs shut down. The victim is left speechless, unable to move, incontinent, and alive (?). More than a quarter of a million American men and women die of stroke each year; perhaps twice as many—half a million—live the last years of their lives substantially crippled and unable to enjoy the retirement for which they worked so long. How's that for an image while you sink your teeth into a tender, juicy, fat steak?

Atherosclerosis can also narrow the channels of your coronary arteries. These are two sets of blood vessels that sit on top of your heart like a crown of tree branches, hence the name "coronary," after their crownlike appearance. There are many "twigs" leading from the branches of coronary arteries; these twigs burrow back into the heart muscle to feed the great pump with fresh, oxygen-carrying blood. Thus, while gallons of fresh blood pass each hour through the inner chambers of the heart, it is the coronary arteries that bring nourishing blood and oxygen to individual muscle fibers within the meaty and business end of the pump.

As atherosclerosis piles up substances in the coronaries, the passageways narrow, reducing blood flow into the heart muscle. Beyond a certain point, the muscle must literally gasp for air, and in so doing causes a great surge of pain, among the worst known to man, angina (from the Latin *angere* meaning "to choke." It is well named). Angina warns the body to take some of the work-load off the heart and temporarily reduce the heart's need for oxygenated blood. For some victims, angina never goes away. For them, even lying in bed may be too much for the heart. Even if it does not incapacitate, angina can, like a stroke, make your later years unbearable, if only because you will be constantly anticipating that stab of strangling pain.

Heart Attack

Most people do not know they have atherosclerosis. Heart attack hangs like a sword over these unwitting victims. It has been discovered in soldiers dying of war injury at as young an age as nineteen. As atherosclerosis progressively clogs the coronaries, one or both of them may close down partially or entirely, in the same way as the brain arteries do in stroke. Coronary-artery shutdown can be the result of a blood clot on the roughened arterial lining, or of a muscle spasm in the artery wall—a cramp—that shuts a narrowed vessel. (Cramps are of no consequence if the channel is wide open.) In either case, blood to a portion of the heart stops—sometimes temporarily, sometimes permanently. A stonemason slams his hammer down on your chest. You suffer angina to the nth power and your heart attack is on.

Survival depends on many factors. If the blood stoppage lasts longer than fifteen minutes, muscle cells will die. If too much of the heart dies, there may not be enough viable heart muscle left to push blood through your body. Blood pressure drops, your kidneys go out of commission, waste products pile up in your body, the weakened heart beats faster but with less efficiency, and finally the heart and brain simply stop working. Death.

Sometimes only a small portion of the heart is affected, but the assault sets off an electrical storm in the heart muscle so that it loses its pumping rhythm. While still healthy, the muscle flaps helplessly, like a wet flag in a mild breeze. No blood moves. The brain cells die. Death.

Or the damage may be intermediate, leaving a weakened heart that can barely keep enough blood moving around the body to feed the various organs. The kidney, for example, becomes inefficient. Water begins to pile up in the tissues and the heart has to work harder. The overworked remnant muscle cannot keep up with demand and grows steadily weaker. Often the victim is left bedridden or at least weak and scared. It may take a few months or a few years, but the heart does eventually give up. Frequently, there is another heart attack as another portion of the coronary system shuts down. Death.

Fortunately, not every heart attack ends in immediate death or incapacity. During the years atherosclerosis has been obliterating your coronary arteries, other blood vessels near the heart muscle, responding to some mysterious chemical agent emitted by the heart, grow tiny new branches that reach out and imbed themselves into the heart muscle to feed it fresh blood. However, these auxiliary blood vessels may take years to grow to full bloom. Imagine, then, a race between the steadily constricting coronary arteries and the burgeoning relief system. As one set of blood vessels grows progressively useless, the other takes over. If you are unlucky and the coronary arteries narrow faster than the relief system develops, the chances are you will have a heart attack—perhaps a fatal one—in your forties or early fifties. If the relief system builds up faster, that attack may be postponed or perhaps never occur. The trick is to slow down the process of atherosclerosis. That is why you need to know about food and how to control it.

If you are an American male, the chances are that your coronary arteries are already partially stuffed (even at the age of nineteen). If you are an American female, you also probably have atherosclerosis, but to a lesser degree than a male of the same age. Overall, men are perhaps four times as susceptible as women. For men, heart-attack danger begins to rise sharply in the late thirties and peaks by the age of sixty. The risk then falls off, reaching a low at age seventy. The age pattern probably reflects the race between the narrowing arteries and the growing relief system. It also tells us that coronary disease kills off susceptible men early, leaving the durable ones.

Women may owe their lower risk to the female sex hormones— the estrogens. In experiments with animals the development of scaly arteries has been retarded through the administering of estrogens. In men, the introduction of estrogens reduces risk of heart attack, but not without inducing large breasts, a high-pitched voice, and a weakening of the male libido—feminizing effects that most men would consider far more threatening than a heart attack.

The increase in coronary-attack risk for women comes ten years later than it does for men, that is, by the mid-forties, when estrogen production begins to slacken. The danger reaches a peak by age seventy. After menopause, when estrogen production has dropped away, a woman's risk of heart attack, kidney disease, and stroke just about equals that of men. Although normally thought of as a man's disease, atherosclerosis takes a heavy toll among women. It happens later, to be sure, but it happens. Women have every reason to be just as concerned about reducing risk as men—in fact, women often suffer more. There is some evidence that atherosclerosis progresses in women at only a slightly slower pace than in men.

If you do have a heart attack, the chances are 1 in 3 that the first one will kill you (the first attack is more lethal for women than for men). Further, the odds are greater than 50-50 that if the attack is lethal, death will come on the same day; you will never get your toes inside the front door of a hospital. I present this data by way of demonstrating the futility of relying primarily on medical treatment to keep a coronary attack from destroying your life. I will go further. If in the back of your mind you are counting on the magnificent medical apparatus that we have in America to return you to mint condition after the attack, forget it. Even with the most elegant coronary-care unit, round-the-clock nursing, electronic wizardry, and superdrugs, the doctor can do little to save your life, that is, add years, reduce incapacity, or remove the possibility—with its accompanying anxiety—that within two to five years you will have another attack that will kill you. Your survival depends largely on the condition of your arteries—the coronaries and the relief system—at the time of the attack and, to some extent, on how successful you are in changing your life style after the attack.

I do not mean to say that you should avoid doctors. Hardly. Under the best circumstances, they can increase your chances of survival six weeks after the attack by about 15 per cent. If you are lucky and have only an electrical-disturbance attack, fast action by a doctor to get your heart beating regularly again means a lot, because in such cases the heart remains relatively undamaged. Survival could mean a long life. What I do want to stress is that medical efforts after an attack do not return you to top condition.

Eating for Protection

Atherosclerosis accounts for half of all deaths. If you can delay the disease, you have an excellent chance of living healthier longer. By now you have begun to suspect, I am sure, that what you eat plays a significant part in the development of the disease. I have been trying to give you motivation for food control by dwelling on atherosclerosis—but there are other reasons for confining your eating to nutritional foods. The proper amounts of vitamins, minerals, and proteins keep resistance to infection high, and prevent premature births and intellectual impairment in children.

It is important also to realize that poor eating is not the sole cause of atherosclerosis. The disease is not a simple process; if it were, science would have conquered it long ago. But most people are used to thinking of a disease as having a single cause (they hope and believe science will find The Cause of cancer, The Cause of heart disease, The Cause of schizophrenia), principally because of their familiarity with the infectious diseases: tuberculosis produced by a bacterium, chickenpox by a virus, syphilis by a spirochete. These have been brought under control, and the habit of thought lingers.

But our modern life-shortening ailments have many causes and pertinent factors, which make them all the harder to understand and control. One such pertinent factor in atherosclerosis is heredity. Scientists are quite sure that if your father, mother, brother, or sister had or has the disease, you have a higher chance of having it. My father died of coronary attack and my brother recovered from one; thus statistically I am a prime target. The figures show that if one of your parents or grandparents died of atherosclerosis—heart attack, angina, stroke—before the age of sixty, your risk is twice as great as for the fellow without such a family tree; if a brother or sister also had or has the ailment, your risk is four times greater than average. Absence of atherosclerosis in your family history provides no absolute insurance against your having it. Your risk is only lower, not zero.

It is a less than comforting picture. But heredity—despite what you may have heard—is not unmanageable. A hereditary factor is operative within a specific environment; when the environment changes, the relevance of the factor may be lessened. Hereditary nearsightedness—myopia—probably often severely handicapped primitive man as he hunted for food. But today's environment has made myopia simply an inconvenience that can be easily corrected with eyeglasses; it is no longer relevant to survival.

Internal environment also can be changed. Victims of the rare Wilson's disease suffer from an inherited fault of body chemistry that allows excess copper to accumulate in the blood and brain. At high levels, copper poisons the nerves, which leads to symptoms of palsy and severe emotional upset, and to early death. A diet low in copper reduces the symptoms. Recently, scientists discovered a chemical that physically captures copper in the body and leads it out through the kidneys. Combined with a low-copper diet, the treatment can return Wilson's-disease patients to near normal.

In the case of atherosclerosis, the hereditary component is a fault of body chemistry that allows a pile-up of fatty material on the inner surface of the arteries. Scientists are hard at work trying to find a pill that will prevent that accumulation. At this writing, several substances are being tested on a wide scale. The preliminary results are promising, and there is a good chance that, as with Wilson's disease, the pill will work optimally only with a suitable diet. The important thing is that meanwhile, in the absence of such medicine, you can alter your internal environment right now by changing your style of eating.

You have probably heard about quick and easy ways to good health through eating natural and organic foods, strictly pure vegetables, unrefined sugar. Allow me to take care of all such fads by making a general, totally supportable statement based on current scientific evidence: *If you are able to change your eating style so as to provide optimum protection against atherosclerosis, you will provide an optimum diet for your general health.* You will not have to worry about vitamins, minerals, proteins, unrefined sugar, natural foods, organic foods, et cetera. (I know that by making this statement I am going to provoke a host of rebuttals from food faddists, so the rule for writing to me, if you want an answer, is: accompany the letter with reprints from regular scientific journals reporting on actual experiments or controlled observations supporting your point of view.)

There are exceptions to my general statement: some individuals suffer from gout, diabetes, or certain rare diseases requiring special diets. The anti-atherosclerosis eating style (notice I did not say diet) can easily be modified to take care of any special problem. Your physician will tell you what foods should be added or subtracted. In any case, the behavior techniques you will learn in order to change your style to the anti-atherosclerosis pattern can be used to modify your eating for medical reasons. Most physicians who require a patient to eat special diets give him no help beyond handing him a piece of paper showing the prohibited and allowed foods.

The food pattern we will be considering emphasizes low-fat and low-saturated-fat foods (saturated fat is generally of animal origin: beef, lamb, pork, and dairy products). There are scientists who doubt the evidence of the connection between fats and atherosclerosis. Some believe that sugar and carbohydrates (starches) are the culprits. In short, we have a controversy. However, by the end of this chapter I think you will agree that even if fat is not the only criminal substance, you have everything to gain (figuratively!) and little to lose in changing your food pattern to de-emphasize fat.

Optimum Weight

Have you ever noticed how few really old people are fat? Tall, thin men seem to outlive all others. A study of American men and women by American insurance companies, one of the largest ever made, indicates that every pound of weight above the optimum adds a significant risk of early death. A man of medium frame, 5 feet 11 inches tall, should weigh 159 pounds (see desirable-weight charts below). If he actually weighs 191 pounds, he has doubled his risk of dying early from atherosclerosis, diabetes, or high blood pressure.

Desirable Weights for Men in Stocking Feet,
Pants, and Shirt (without Jacket or Vest) *

HEIGHT		FRAME		
Feet	*Inches*	*Small*	*Medium*	*Large*
5	1	113	121	131
5	2	116	124	134
5	3	119	127	137
5	4	122	130	140
5	5	126	134	144
5	6	130	138	149
5	7	134	142	154
5	8	138	146	158
5	9	142	150	162
5	10	146	155	166
5	11	150	159	171
6	0	154	164	176
6	1	159	168	181
6	2	163	173	186
6	3	167	178	191

Note: Nude weight is between 2 and 3 pounds less than this table indicates. For heights above 6 feet 3 inches add 5 pounds for each inch.

Desirable Weights for Women in Stocking Feet, Light Dress (No Heavy Skirts, Suits or Jackets)

HEIGHT		FRAME		
Feet	*Inches*	*Small*	*Medium*	*Large*
4	8	94	101	111
4	9	97	103	113
4	10	99	106	116
4	11	102	109	119
5	0	105	112	122
5	1	108	115	125
5	2	111	119	129
5	3	114	123	133
5	4	118	127	137
5	5	122	131	141
5	6	126	135	145
5	7	130	139	149
5	8	134	143	153
5	9	138	147	158
5	10	142	151	162

Note: Nude weight is between 2 and 3 pounds less than this table indicates. For heights above 5 feet 10 inches add 4 pounds for each inch.
* Based on Metropolitan Life Insurance Company's Table of Desirable Weights, modified by M. B. Glenn in *Clinical Nutrition*, by Norman Jolliffe (New York: Harper & Row, 1972).

Weight-and-height tables used to give *average* weights for individuals. Now they give *optimum*, or *desired*, weights. The desired weight is that poundage at which you have the lowest risk of early death. Desired weights are uniformly about fifteen pounds under the average weight for men, about twelve pounds for women. In terms of risk of early death, America is an overweight nation. "Pure" overweight is not as lethal as overweight complicated by other factors. Recent studies show that overweight plus some other infirmity spells a higher risk than overweight alone. However, it is a rare person who is purely overweight, without a complicating factor like high blood pressure, a family history of atherosclerosis, a sedentary life, or high levels of cholesterol in his blood.

The Cholesterol Conundrum

Ah, cholesterol. The magic word. The confusing word. You have probably heard that a) cholesterol is bad for you, b) cholesterol doesn't matter, or c) cholesterol is good for you, or all three. First, what is cholesterol? A chemical found naturally in all animal tissues . . . in your muscles, brains, liver, et cetera. It is not a fat, although, because it is so closely allied with the process by which your body uses fat, it has been confused with it. You eat cholesterol when you eat animal products; you also eat fat when you eat animal products. Some foods have large amounts of both cholesterol and fat: eggs, beef, brains. Some have substantial amounts of cholesterol but low amounts of fat: shrimp, lobster, and other shellfish. Some foods have large amounts of fat but little cholesterol: cream, ice cream, hard cheese. Is cholesterol good for you?

You must have cholesterol; it is essential to the operation of the human chemical machine, which produces hormones, among other substances. Your body, mostly the liver, manufactures cholesterol. Without it, you would die. In this sense, cholesterol is good for you.

On the other hand, if you have too much cholesterol circulating in your body, it will begin to stick to the walls of your arteries— an effect noted by two Russian scientists back in 1905. But the overabundance of cholesterol in the blood as a factor in atherosclerosis is currently the best-documented story. You acquire too much cholesterol either because you eat too much beef, eggs, and other high-cholesterol foods, or because your body manufactures more than you need.

Some people produce cholesterol in very large amounts because they have an inherited tendency, which is, incidentally, rare. Predictably, such persons have heart attacks early in life from atherosclerosis. Another—much more common—reason for excess cholesterol is that the body is overstimulated to produce it. Overstimulation occurs with eating—not cholesterol but fats, and in particular animal fats: beef, dairy products, pork, and lamb. Most scientists would agree that eating animal fats is a much more powerful factor in increasing the amount of cholesterol in your body than the amount of cholesterol you eat.

There is another, somewhat confusing fact: eating large amounts of cholesterol does increase the cholesterol in the blood, but not by as much as you might think. Unfortunately, there is no easy way to find out how much cholesterol is circulating in your body. The measurement must be made in a laboratory from a sample of your blood. If you are going to reduce the cholesterol in your blood by changing your food pattern, it will be a good idea to check on how well you are doing. In some states it is a simple matter of going to a medical laboratory and asking for a cholesterol check. In other states only a physician can order the test. What he will usually tell you is that your cholesterol is "all right" or "average."

Unfortunately, average cholesterol, like average weight, is too high. Scientists measure the amount of cholesterol in your blood in milligrams, but it is easier to think of it as a cholesterol score. The average American male score lies between 220 and 240. The average Japanese male has a score under 200. American men are dying 1.7 times faster than Japanese men, that is, at a 70 per cent higher rate; most of that difference is accounted for by a higher prevalance of atherosclerosis in the Americans. If your score is higher than 260—about one-third of American men are in that category—your risk of dying of heart attack is more than four times as great as that of the average Japanese or of the American male who has a cholesterol score under 200.

So what you want to know from your doctor or from the laboratory is the actual number. I am puzzled as to why doctors hesitate to educate their patients about this number. Certainly they have no compunction about weight numbers, so why not cholesterol numbers? If I had my way, I would make cholesterol measurements available at minimal cost to anyone wanting them. Right now the price is about ten dollars—cheap for what you get out of it, yet a deterrent to having it done, especially when you are not yet sick.

Without turning this into a scientific treatise with footnotes and citations, I will make the following statements, for which—take me at my word—there exists extensive scientific evidence (these apply to women as well as men, although the effects are not as pronounced, nor do they occur as early as they do for men):

1. Populations that have high blood-cholesterol scores—American, Australian, British—have high risk of atherosclerosis with the consequent heart attack, angina, and stroke.

2. Populations that have low blood-cholesterol scores—Japanese, Italian—have low risk of atherosclerosis.

3. Populations that eat diets high in animal fat (beef, lamb, pork, dairy products) have high blood cholesterol and high risk of atherosclerosis. Conversely, populations that eat diets low in animal fat (mostly vegetables and fish) have low blood-cholesterol scores and low risk of atherosclerosis.

4. It has been demonstrated that changing an eating pattern so that it is low in animal fat and cholesterol results in reduction of the blood-cholesterol score.

As of this writing, the most important ingredients in raising cholesterol levels are animal fats, which stimulate the cholesterol factory in your body to work overtime, and foods containing cholesterol. But if you change your eating style, throttle back on cholesterol production and absorption, what are your chances of reducing risk of atherosclerosis?

Scientists are desperately struggling with this puzzle. As you can imagine, an unequivocal demonstration proving that decreased animal fat and cholesterol in food resulted in longer life would touch off a massive food-education campaign; new laws would be passed governing the production of food—cattle, sheep, and pigs would be raised lean, butter would be eliminated, milk would have little or no cream. Fish and fowl would become the order of the day. But the definitive experiment has yet to be done. One group of scientists has proposed that fifty thousand men be enrolled in a massive test of the low-fat diet as protection against atherosclerosis. Half would eat the regular American diet, the other half a special low-fat diet. The two groups would then be compared for heart-attack rate. But only part of the experiment has been done. The major test has not been approved or funded. Estimates put the cost between $100 million and $300 million over a ten-year period. It is a sad comment on our times that no approval can be obtained for an experiment that could add from four to eight years of life to the average man during his most productive years. Yet the maximum cost is less (by about $500 million) than the cost of a new door on the fire-stricken Apollo moonship or one-half of 1 per cent of our annual defense budget. Put another way, the investment amounts to five cents per American per year.

Nevertheless, scientists have proceeded with less-than-airtight trials. Two were conducted in male institutions, two among men living at home. In each of the four, half the men received a diet high in animal fat, the others a diet low in animal fat. The men on low-animal-fat foods in all four tests showed a reduction in blood cholesterol and in signs and symptoms of atherosclerosis; those who had started with the highest cholesterol scores achieved the greatest reduction in their scores—and the greatest reduction in heart-attack risk. It is never too late to start; even if you have gobs of the stuff in your blood, you can cut it down.

But some scientists say it is too early to recommend that all Americans change their eating style; not enough is known to make the judgment. Such a position reminds me of a true story. Perhaps it will help you to make up your mind.

In the time of the great cholera epidemics in London in the 1840's and 1850's, there lived a doctor named John Snow, physician to Queen Victoria. More than a court dandy, Snow was a scientist. Observing that the incidence of cholera seemed to be concentrated only in areas of London served by certain water supplies, he decided to follow through on the possibility that water carried the disease. His next step was to place a pin on a map of London for every case reported in the epidemic of 1854. The pins clustered around the Broad Street well. (One pin represented a lady who lived some distance away from the well. He found out that as a child she had lived in the Broad Street neighborhood. Now, years later, she somehow got the idea that the Broad Street well of her childhood produced water that had curative powers. She had a pint of it brought to her home every day—and she came down with cholera.)

Snow removed the handle of the Broad Street pump and the epidemic subsided. He did this before Pasteur had articulated his germ theory of disease, before the cholera germ was discovered, and before water-borne infection was a proven process. Strictly speaking, I suppose Snow acted rashly—he did not have all the data, did not know the "real cause" of cholera, and he operated on only "statistical" evidence. But then, he did stop the epidemic. Perhaps it is time to remove the handle on the cholesterol pump—animal fats.

What Are Your Odds?

If you want to get some idea of what your odds are for suffering a coronary earlier than your fellow Americans, just take the following simple survival test:

1. Look at the desirable-weight tables; are you 15 per cent or more overweight?

_____ Yes   _____ No

(If your arithmetic is rotten and you cannot figure per cents, first find your weight in the table and check the height that goes with it. If that height is five or more inches taller than you are, you are 15 per cent overweight.)

2. Is your cholesterol score 220 or above?

_____ Yes   _____ No

3. Did your grandparents, parents, brothers, or sisters have a heart attack, stroke, angina, or other form of hardening of the arteries before the age of sixty?

_____ Yes   _____ No

4. Have you or has any other close member of your family had a diagnosis of gout or diabetes?

_____ Yes   _____ No

5. Have you had a heart attack, stroke, or other form of hardening of the arteries?

_____ Yes   _____ No

6. Do you smoke two or more packs of cigarettes a day?

_____ Yes   _____ No

7. Are you a sedentary person?

_____ Yes   _____ No

If you answered yes to any single question, then your risk of heart attack is twice that of the person who answers no to all the questions. A yes to questions 1 through 5 means you are a candidate for diet change. If you answered yes to question 6 or 7 and no to all others, you may not have to change your diet (but you should do something about smoking or exercise).

If you answered yes to any two questions, your risk approximately doubles. Three yeses doubles the risk once more, making the odds 8 to 1 that you will have a heart attack before the average naysayer.

It is hard to say exactly how much your life will be shortened by a yes or a combination of yeses. Having had one heart attack is more life-shortening than smoking two packs of cigarettes a day, which is more life-shortening than high blood cholesterol, which is more risky than overweight, and so on. And some combinations are deadlier than others—for example, cigarette-smoking plus a family history of heart disease.

However, here are my guesses at the life-shortening properties of your habits. One yes means you have a 50-50 chance of shortening your life by about four years (the range is from two years, for lack of exercise, to eight years, for smoking). In other words, your odds are even that you will die before reaching the average life expectancy: for men, sixty-eight years; for women, seventy-two years.

If you answered yes twice, your life may be shortened by as much as six years, with a range of four to ten years. If you answered yes three times, life-shortening may average eight years, with a range of six to twelve years. A three-yes man has a 50-50 chance of losing eight years, one chance in four of dying in his fifties, and one chance in eight of dying in his forties.

Odds on Surviving to a Given Age, Based on Yeses and Noes to the Survival Test Taken by a Twenty-five-year-old Man

	ODDS			
	1/2	*1/4*	*1/8*	
All noes	71	66	61	
1 yes	67	61	57	Surviving Age
2 yeses	64	59	53	
3 yeses	62	54	49	

The figures are based on my guesses at the odds of surviving your habits. A bad combination of three yeses could make the last figure in the last column 47. Similar figures apply for women, but five years later.

I can make these odds somewhat more graphic: suppose somebody offered you $100,000 to stand before a man with a gun and allow him to shoot at you from a distance of one hundred yards. You are told that on the average he hits his target one out of eight times. He has one bullet. Would you take the chance?

There are only odds, no certainties at all. Is it worth changing your pattern of life to change the odds? That's up to you.

Where to Start

Start with overweight. Before checking the desirable-weight charts, you should get a good idea of your frame size. One way of doing that is to place your thumb and forefinger (the pointing finger) of one hand around the wrist of the other. If the gap between the two fingers measures more than one-quarter of an inch, you have a large frame; if the fingers just touch, you have a medium frame; if they overlap, you have a small frame.

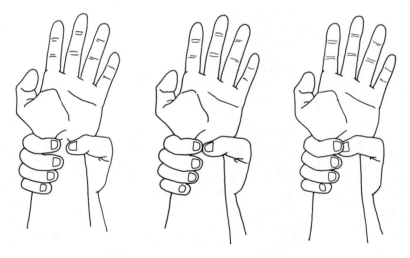

Another method of estimating the type of frame you have is to check your shoe size; the size of your feet is a good indicator of your bony structure.

Frame Size

	Small	Medium	Large
Men's shoe size	under 8	8 or 9	over 9
Women's shoe size	under 6	6 or 7	over 7

Sometimes there's a conflict between the two methods. My wife, who is just under five feet tall, wears a size five shoe and is therefore small frame by shoe size, but she is large frame by the wrist test. I would go by the test that gives the smaller frame. That will indicate a lower optimum weight, which is almost always a safer goal (and incidentally, in my view, will make you look better).

Another way to determine whether or not you are overweight is to grab a pinch of skin just under the last rib on your right side with thumb and forefinger. If there is more than an inch of thickness, you are overweight. (No fair pinching hard.) Or try this: lie down on your back on the floor, nude. Place a yardstick along the line of your body so that it touches the lower part of the breastbone and the pubic bone (the bone just north of your genital area). If your belly sticks up in the middle and prevents the stick from touching either bone, you are overweight.

If by the chart you are overweight and yet not so by the pinch or ruler tests, you may have your weight in muscle instead of fat. I would then subtract five pounds from your weight and check the chart again. Most people are overweight by about 15 per cent. When confronted by the desirable-weight charts, the chubby one is heard to cry "My God! That can't be true. I'd be a freak if I weighed that little. I would look sick."

Well, that is exactly the idea. I know one physician, with a morbid sense of humor, who says you should lose weight until your friends think you have cancer. We have become so used to identifying average with healthy that when we see somebody who is of optimal weight, we immediately think something is wrong. When I was thirty years old, I weighed 190 pounds. For a man with a large frame, 5 feet 10 inches tall, that is 15 per cent overweight. When I began to lose weight, my mother thought I had some terrible disease that I was keeping secret from her.

The depressing fact is that as we grow older we get fatter. Many people believe that being heavier with age is okay, if not desirable. It isn't. If you are nice and trim and in your early twenties, you should try to look that way for the next six decades. Not only will you draw admiration; you will also be improving your chances of *living* those next sixty years.

Mesomorphs and Such

Tall, skinny guys live longest; short, fat ones die early. This statement summarizes a body of data concerning the connection between early death and type of physique. The matter is controversial. However, it does serve as a warning to those of us who are of the "wrong" body type.

Which is the wrong type? Scientists have divided physiques into three basic categories: ectomorph, mesomorph, and endomorph. Ectomorphs are skinny. By the wrist test, they end up being small frame. Endomorphs are fat, but they too end up being small frame by the wrist test. Mesomorphs are muscular, heavy set, and large or medium frame by the wrist test. They are the type most vulnerable to heart attack. Endomorphs may be examples of pure overweight. (But don't count on that; it takes somewhat of an expert to decide differences between endomorphs and mesomorphs.)

In any case, if you are large frame and relatively short, overweight may be more dangerous for you than for any other body type. Mesomorphs: lose weight!

The Arithmetic of Weight Gain

You gain weight because you take in more food energy than your body uses. You lose weight because you use more energy than you take in by way of food. You maintain an even weight if the energy you take in through food is the same as the energy you expend. It's that simple. You don't need any other explanation. It is thus impossible to believe statements like: "I eat nothing at all and I still gain weight"; "Listen. I eat half of what I used to and I don't lose a pound."

The only way to lose weight is to make sure your food intake is below what you need to keep up your daily activities. There is no other way. You can do this by simply decreasing your food intake, or you can continue at your present eating level and increase your activities, thus raising your energy output above energy intake. The latter is of course the harder of the two.

Food energy is measured in calories, a familiar word. The low-calorie-food craze has paid off handsomely for a significant part of the food industry, but unfortunately the calorie concept has been applied in so helter-skelter a fashion that we are left with a host of misconceptions and myths. So let's get the calorie story straight.

Your body needs energy to do its work, to move your arms and legs, digest food, keep warm, and carry out the complex chemical reactions that are life itself. That energy comes from one source: food. We are not like plants; we cannot turn our faces to the sun and absorb energy. And we cannot manufacture energy inside our bodies. Energy cannot be created or destroyed, but it can be transformed: chemical energy in food becomes the electrical energy of our nerves, the mechanical energy of muscle contraction, and heat. All that energy is measured in calories. As you lie abed doing nothing, you are using up calories of energy just to keep the machinery idling. If you chop wood, you expend additional calories. The balance is an equation representing a body in energy:

energy (calories) used = energy (calories) eaten as food

The body does not throw away excess calories; it stores them for future use. This was a wonderful lifesaving mechanism for the primitive hunter, who didn't know when he was going to get his next meal. In modern times, we don't need such an efficient storage system. When we overeat it would be nice if those extra calories were stored for only a few hours. Instead they are stored, as fat, for months, even years, depending on how much and how long we overeat. Fat has the highest caloric content per pound of any body tissue: 3,500 calories, compared with 1,400 calories per pound each for sugar and protein. If you overeat, the difference between what you take in and what you use is stored as fat:

calories in − calories used = calories stored as fat

As far as anybody knows, there is no way of getting around this equation. Some rare individuals—perhaps one person in a thousand—have a glandular disturbance that diverts calories preferentially to fat at the expense of other bodily functions. However, do not use this as an excuse for gaining weight "no matter how little I eat." You probably do not have this ailment, and even if you do, the diversion of calories to fat can be overcome by reducing intake still further.

Let's see what happens if you eat just a few more calories each day than your body uses. Suppose you burn up 2,400 calories a day and you eat 2,600 calories of food. The difference is 200 calories, or the amount of energy in two thinly buttered slices of bread. That means you are storing 200 calories as .06 pounds of fat, or one ounce. It doesn't look like much. But suppose your weight when you began adding those 200 calories to your daily intake was 120 pounds. Look what happens in one year:

$$365 \times .06 = 22 \text{ lbs.}$$

So there you have it. By eating only 200 calories more each day than you need—a Coke, half a slice of pizza, an ice-cream cone—you end up gaining twenty-two pounds in a year, forty-four in two years. Actually, the gain would not adhere quite that closely to the formula, since the body would need more energy to carry the extra pounds around. So if you kept your daily caloric intake at 2,600 calories your weight would level off in a few months, regardless of your height, to about 155 pounds if you are moderately active at middle age.

Because of a marvelous mechanism the body has for regulating its food intake, few people actually count the calories going into their mouths. Fewer still can keep track accurately of what they take in, because individual portions may be more caloric or less than can be estimated. A person who keeps his weight within a pound or two year after year is actually keeping his daily caloric intake within a 10- or 20-calorie daily fluctuation. If he eats about 2,000 calories a day, his unconscious caloric balancing is accurate to within a fraction of 1 per cent, which is more accurate than most scientific instruments.

How does the body do it? Very little is known about the appetite mechanism responsible for such fine controls. Scientists have found that damage to certain parts of the brain unleashes a voracious appetite. And that is only one part of the carefully balanced complex chemical mechanism that makes use of a large amount of data—such as total fat stored away, the number of fat cells, the amount of sugar in the blood, the last time the stomach was full, the time of day, the taste of food, the amount of exercise the body does, the day-by-day emotional stress, eating speed, and the ethnically learned eating style—to regulate caloric intake every day. Incredible, isn't it? Yet it is possible consciously to orchestrate all these elements by a training program using reward and punishment.

What Makes Weight Loss Happen

To lose weight, you simply have to use more calories than you take in. To make up the energy deficit, your body calls on its fat deposits. Suppose your daily caloric use is 2,600 calories—the energy you burn up—and you take in only 2,400 calories. That gives you a *200-calorie daily deficit*. So you're burning up .06 pounds of your stored fat every day. Again, while it doesn't seem like much, if you keep it up for 365 days you get a weight loss of twenty-two pounds, forty-four pounds in two years! Imagine, just by giving up the equivalent of two slices of bread each day, you end up losing twenty-two pounds a year.

Ah, but there is a catch to all this. Two catches, in fact. For one thing, it is almost impossible for you, practically or consciously, to measure out the amount of food you eat accurately enough so that you can maintain a 200-calorie deficit. Imagine trying to figure out the calorie content of a slice of restaurant meat loaf. Then, too, there is the fact that a lighter body does not use as much energy as an overweight one; even the heart needs less energy because there is less tissue to be serviced. If you kept your calorie intake at 2,400 calories, you would lose pounds until your weight would require just 2,400 calories. Obviously, it is necessary to keep track of the food you eat so that you can sustain the food pattern long enough to lose weight, eating just the amount of food that will create a calorie deficit.

In order to change your style of eating so that it will be effective, you must sustain the new behavior over a long enough time to make the new behavior automatic—beyond your conscious control. That is, you have to make the new pattern into a habit. The longer you persisted in your old eating habits and found them rewarding, the longer it will take to modify your style permanently. Yes, there is quick weight loss, but to achieve it you must cut your food intake by more than 1,000 calories a day. For a person who has been living on, say, 2,700 calories daily, such a cutback may be pure misery. Further, the grotesqueness of the eating pattern will make it impossible to maintain after the desired amount of weight is lost. The fundamental idea is to lose weight by styling your pattern close to the way you want to eat for the rest of your life. Although I do not have substantial evidence for it, my feeling is that it takes at least ten weeks to retrain your eating pattern. It is much tougher to sustain behavior control over a longer period, but the pay-off is bigger: permanent change of eating pattern, permanent weight loss.

If you are 15 per cent overweight, you should aim at losing between a pound and a pound and a half a week. If you are more than 15 per cent overweight, you can lose between two and three pounds a week, but not more. In the first case, that is a deficit of between 500 and 800 calories a day; in the second, between 1,000 and 1,500 calories a day. Individuals who are more than 15 per cent overweight usually need outside help for motivation.

For reducing your daily consumption of calories, there are at least three good methods to choose from: a general restriction of foods, following a menu plan, and counting calories. Let's look at all three.

Restriction of Food Intake

Unless you go about it systematically, you are likely to forget which foods you are restricting and your diet will subtly shift to high-calorie foods without your conscious knowledge. I suggest a systematic restriction of foods by class, that is, according to the amount of food energy they contain. Easy, eh? Dr. H. M. Whyte has developed a helpful chart (see next page). Each day takes *two*

The order of placement in the food columns indicates the relative richness in calories of average servings of the different items. Nutritional needs are met if the daily diet includes two normal servings of food from each of the first five columns. To get down to your desirable weight move *down* the food columns, move *up* the exercise column. It is not necessary to count calories. No

CALORIES GAINED FROM COMMON SERVINGS

	Dairy Group	Meat Group	Vegetables	Fruit
4—		Pork, goose		
3½—		Lamb, mutton, duck		
3—		Beef, turkey		
2½—		Sausages (2)		
		Ham		
2—		Veal, cold cuts tongues, nuts (¼ cup) fatty fish (salmon, herring, mackerel, shad)		
1½—	Whole milk (1 cup)	Chicken, crab, lobster		Avocado (½) Dried fruits
1—	Ice cream (4 tb.) Cream (2 tb.) Cheese (1″ cube) Butter (1 tb.) Skim milk (1 cup) Egg, whole Egg yolk	Fish, oysters (6) Shrimp (½ lb.) Bacon, fried (2 strips) Brains, tripe	Sweet potato Lentils Potatoes, artichokes, sweet corn	Banana Canned fruits Other fruit
½—	Cottage cheese Egg white Whole milk (1 tb.)		Mushrooms and other vegetables	Pineapple (2 sl.) Melon Tomato Strawberries (6)
0—			Lettuce, cucumber, squash, marrow	

Calorie Units (left vertical label)

Note: Each calorie unit is approx. 100 calories. Common average servings are meant—e.g., 3 or

* From *Eat to Your Heart's Content* by H. M. Whyte (New York: Hawthorn Books, 1972). Used

food is forbidden, but the selection of a calorie-rich item should be compensated for at other meals. Don't skip meals. Weigh weekly on the same scales, and in the same clothes. A satisfactory rate of loss is 1 to 2 lbs. per week. If this is not achieved, eat still less, exercise more.

			CALORIES SPENT IN 30 MINUTES OF	
Cereals	Fluids	Extra Foods	Exercise	
				—4
				—3½
		Pie	Chopping, loading,	—3
		Hamburger	tennis, skiing, climbing	
		Sandwich (2 slices average filling)		—2½
	Flavored whole milk	Waffle, spaghetti, macaroni, rice	Shoveling, sawing, swimming, cycling	
		Scrambled egg	Tennis	—2
Oatmeal	Whole milk (1 cup)	Cake, chocolate (1 oz.)	Walking, dancing, golf, gardening	—1½
Breakfast cereals	Beer, wine	⎧ Cooking fat, lard, oil (1 tb.)	Domestic chores,	
Bread (1 slice)	spirits (glass or nip)	⎨ Pancakes (2)	bowling, baseball	
		⎩ Caramels, etc. (1 oz.)		—1
		⎧ Butter, margarine (1 tb.)		
		⎨ Mayonnaise (1 tb.)		
		⎩ Biscuits (1 oz.)		
Crackers		Peanut butter (1 tb.)		
	⎧ Soft drink (8 oz.)	Tomato sauce (2 tb.)	Process work, dressing, shaving, washing	
	⎨ Thick soup		Clerical work, sewing	
	⎪ Fruit juice (4 oz.)	Syrup, honey, jam (1 tb.)	Sitting (watching TV!)	—½
	⎩ Tomato juice (4 oz.)	Flour (1 tb.), sugar (2 ts.)	Sleeping	
	Thin soup	Cocoa (1 ts.)		
	Water	Saccharine		—0
	Black coffee and tea			

Calorie Units (right-hand axis label)

4 oz. of meats, 1 cup of oatmeal, 2 apricots, small bunch of grapes, slice of melon, etc.

with permission.

portions from each of the first five columns—that's ten portions spread over three meals. You may add a portion or two from columns 6 and 7. Try to keep moving down the food columns, that is, select foods of lower caloric value, and up the exercise column. Notice that thirty minutes of walking equals the calorie equivalent of a cup of whole milk. If you take a rich food from the upper part of one column in one meal, take another food from the bottom of the same column at another meal. No seconds!

Dr. Whyte has considerably simplified the problem of keeping track of food intake, but it will avail you little unless you simultaneously apply behavior-control methods, with which you are already familiar. In Dr. Whyte's scheme, you have the choice in each column to select a food high up or at the bottom. That is when you apply behavior control. If you are in a cafeteria and your eyes linger on the pork, go through the punishment-reward sequence to avoid selecting it. As your selection of foods from the lower portions of the columns becomes more and more consistent, your new eating pattern gets closer to being automatic. Eventually you will forget about columns, rewards, and punishments. You will have achieved desirable weight and you will be able to maintain it.

Above all, to ensure that behavior control in conjunction with Dr. Whyte's scheme will work, use the Jolliffe self-monitoring chart discussed in chapter 6. It provides the best way of checking whether you are losing weight at just the right rate.

If Dr. Whyte's columns do not appeal to you, there are other, albeit less accurate, ways of restricting your food intake. The no-no/yes-yes list is a variant of Dr. Whyte's columns. As you will notice, it shows foods in order of their caloric richness; they are also listed according to their saturated-fat content. If you combine this list with the rules of the Prudent Diet (discussed later on in this chapter), you will end up with a varied, low-saturated-fat, low-calorie eating pattern.

You should avoid the foods in the first column, which I have labeled NEVER. If you have something from the first column twice a week, it is just about enough. So NEVER means "hardly ever." You can have something from the second column once a day, from the third twice a day, and something from the fourth column at every meal. You can copy the list onto a small index card and carry it with you, both as a reminder and for use as a punishment device in your behavior-control program. The no-no/ yes-yes chart will help you keep track of food; the behavior-control method will enable you to change your habits; the self-monitoring charts keep track of your progress.

Never (No-No) *(Hardly Ever)*	*Sometimes* *(No-Yes)*	*Usually* *(Yes-No)*	*Always* *(Yes-Yes)*
Cake, pie, pastry	Potatoes, rice	Fish	Vegetables
Pancakes, waffles	Spaghetti	Shellfish	Fruit
Whole milk	Macaroni	Chicken	Fruit juices
Butter, cream	Soft drinks	Turkey	Tomato juice
Ice cream	Wine	Veal	Egg white
Hard cheese	Beer	Cottage cheese	Vegetables
Cream cheese	Liquor	Skim milk	juices
Egg yolk	Candy	Bread	
Beef, lamb	Angel food cake	Cereal	
Pork, ham, bacon		Margarine	
Sausages		Gelatin dessert	
Sauces			

Note: Keep the selections varied and remember that dishes made with more than one food count according to each ingredient.

Still another restricting technique was suggested to me by my fellow science writer, Robert Goldman—who lost forty pounds and kept them off. He suggests leaving at least one-third of each normal portion on your plate (if you are clearheaded about what you are trying to do, you won't compensate by taking larger portions). This method is an especially apt one for practicing behavior modification. As you have learned, the sight of food is a stimulus for eating, and the ability to leave food means that you are effectively countering the stimulus. You counter the stimulus by invoking the usual reward/punishment methods. The food's power to make you eat will decline with every success you have in leaving food on your plate. Take the usual portion, not a smaller one, and leave food uneaten (however much that injures your frugal nature).

Menus

A second general method of reducing calorie intake is to follow daily meal plans. Some people who are well organized find this easy to do. One menu plan I tried was suggested to me by Dr. Jeremiah Stamler, professor of preventive medicine at Northwestern University. I call it the old-fashioned meal; he calls it the continental dinner.

Remember the old-time dinner from soup to nuts? Well, believe it or not, if you modify that dinner it is possible to reduce your caloric total—and have a marvelous meal. Here is a typical one, showing the calorie content of each course:

Clear soup	10 calories
Salad with dressing (1 tbs.)	120
Shrimp cocktail	85
Pasta with low-fat sauce	150
Two medallions of veal, low-fat sauce	200
One green vegetable	15
Fresh fruit cup with kirsch	130
Coffee, tea, or diet drink (no sugar)	10 (if milk added)
Total:	710 calories

If you want a glass of wine, add 100 calories; or if you prefer milk (skim milk, please), add 85 calories; or a slice of bread (no butter), 100 calories.

An evening meal of between 700 and 800 calories is quite moderate for a diet that can be as high as 2,000 calories a day. Of course you can see how this old-fashioned dinner could, with slight changes, easily become a meal of 2,000 calories. Just substitute thick soup for clear, French-fried potatoes for the pasta, an eight-ounce steak for the veal, several slices of bread or rolls for one slice, a couple of bottles of beer for one, and a slice of pie topped with cheese for fruit cup, and your dinner has escalated.

If you follow the Stamler menu every night for dinner with the proper substitutions (see the Prudent Diet guidelines), you can be assured of getting only about 700 calories. Low-calorie substitutes include chicken, turkey, or fish for the veal, potatoes (not mashed with cream) or rice for the pasta, tomato juice for the soup, a gelatin dessert for the fresh fruit. Keep the portions the same as always; if you like, combine this plan with the Goldman idea of leaving something on your plate.

Occasionally you may use pork, beef, or lamb as the meat course, but the portion should be kept small—one pork chop or two thin slices of loin, a small (four-ounce) steak, beef or lamb stew that has been defatted, a thin slice of ham.

The usual restaurant portion is too big by about a third. Steakhouse portions are too big by 100 per cent or more. Therefore, in restaurants plan to leave about half of the meat course on your plate. Behavior-control methods will enable you to do it.

When following the menu plan at home, use behavior control to avoid eating second portions or taking too large a portion, and to resist between-meal and night eating. The latter is especially important: you might eat a well-planned meal of 700 calories and then ruin it by adding another 700 calories "just nibbling."

What Good Breakfast and Lunch Menus Should Include

Breakfast	Calories	Lunch	Calories
Fruit or fruit juice	75	Fruit or fruit juice	75
Bread or cereal (pat of margarine or jam)	100	Bread, 1 slice	75
		†Eggs, fish, fowl, meat, or cottage cheese	200
Skim milk	85		
*Eggs, fish, cottage cheese	150	Green or red vegetable or both	27
Total:	410	Beverage: coffee, tea, no-calorie drink	10 (if you add milk)
		or	
		Skim milk	85
		Total:	470

* One egg, small fish, scoop of cottage cheese; if you must have bacon use the Canadian kind, but not more than once a week.
† Two eggs, small portion of fish or fowl, a thin slice of meat or a 3-ounce hamburger patty (half the usual restaurant size), a large scoop of cottage cheese.

Notice that the Stamler dinner plus the two meals shown above add up to only 1,580 calories, yet achieve a great variety of food.

Portions and calorie counts can often be larger than you realize; allow about 10 per cent more calories, which brings your total close to 1,700. But even on 1,700 calories a day most people will lose weight.

Weight Loss per Week on 1,700 Calories a Day for Normally Active Persons in the Thirty-to-Forty Age Range

Present Weight in Pounds	Pound Loss Per Week	
	Men	*Women*
100	0	.2 (gain)
120	.6	.5
140	1.4	1.0
160	2.0	1.8
180	3.0	2.4

The menus I have laid out work best for people who weigh between 120 and 160 pounds; the weight loss is no greater than two pounds a week. But the menus are probably too rich for people between 100 and 120 pounds, and too lean for those above 160 pounds. For the latter the weight loss is a little too fast. Slight modifications can make the menu plan work for both groups: to reduce the richness, simply eliminate the bread or cereal at breakfast and the kirsch and salad dressing at dinner. To make it less lean, increase the portions somewhat. The Jolliffe chart will tell you if you are on the right track.

Counting Calories

For the mathematically-minded, counting calories is easy. Combined with behavior-control methods, it may be just the right technique for you. Your first task is to set your daily intake at a level that will lose between one and two pounds a week. You can do that by observing the Jolliffe chart for several weeks. Start out by eating 2,000 calories a day for a week and see what happens to your chart. If that is too high, reduce the intake; if too low, increase your eating.

If you're at all good with numbers you can calculate your optimum calorie intake by figuring out your daily calorie needs, using the sample given below. You will need to refer to the tables showing the daily calorie requirements for men and women of normal weight for each decade of life to age eighty (page 175). The tables assume you are engaged in housework, office employment, or operate some light machinery. If you are retired or just sit around most of the time, you need about 10 per cent less than the tables show. If you engage in heavy work, add from 10 per cent to 20 per cent. Add 4 calories for every pound you are overweight. Thus if you are a forty-four-year-old medium-frame man, 5 feet 10 inches tall and weighing 185 pounds, your normal calorie requirement would be 2,560 calories a day plus 120 calories for those thirty extra pounds, a total of 2,680.

Your calculations will look somewhat like an income-tax form or an accountant's balance sheet; they can be accurate within from 5 per cent to 15 per cent, depending on your activity. That's why you need the Jolliffe chart; it guides you when the calculations are off.

In order to give you a short cut to figuring your calorie needs, I have devised the list of multipliers you will find accompanying the figuring-your-calorie-needs sample. I based my calculations on the information in the calorie-requirement tables. Just multiply your present weight by the proper multiplier. Suppose you are a woman, age thirty-three, working as a physical-education teacher, which is considered heavy work. Your multiplier is 18. If you now weigh 125 pounds, multiply 125 by 18, which equals 2,250 calories. That is your daily caloric need at your present weight.

Figuring Out Your Daily Calorie Needs

	Column A	Column B
1. Actual Weight	————	
2. Desirable Weight (see pages 151–152)	————	
3. Difference (No. 1 minus No. 2)	————	————
(Multiply this number by 4 and enter in column B)		

	Column A	Column B
4. Calories at Desirable Weight (see page 175); enter figure in both columns	_____	_____
5. Heavy Worker: take 10% of (4); (enter figure in both columns)	_____	_____

or

	Column A	Column B
6. Very Heavy Worker: take 20% of (4); (enter figure in both columns)	_____	(_____)
7. Retired: take 10% of (4); enter it also in column B as an amount to be SUBTRACTED	_____	(_____)

8. Take the sum of all the figures in column B, being careful to subtract the calories of No. 7 if you are retired

Daily calories needed to maintain present weight _____

Multipliers to Determine Daily Calorie Needs

	AGE						
Men	*15–19*	*20–29*	*30–39*	*40–49*	*50–59*	*60–69*	*70–79*
Normal worker	22	20	17	16	15	14	13
Heavy worker	24	22	19	18	17	15	14
Very heavy worker	26	24	20	19	18	17	16
Retired	20	18	15	14	13	13	12
Women							
Normal worker	19	17	16	15	15	14	13
Heavy worker	21	19	18	17	17	15	14
Very heavy worker	23	20	19	18	18	17	16
Retired	17	15	15	13	13	12	12

Daily Calorie Requirement for Men of Normal Weight*

Height		AGE						
Ft.	In.	15–19	20–29	30–39	40–49	50–59	60–69	70–79
5	1	2,690	2,310	2,160	2,100	2,020	1,750	1,610
5	2	2,750	2,390	2,220	2,110	2,070	1,790	1,650
5	3	2,820	2,450	2,280	2,160	2,110	1,830	1,690
5	4	2,880	2,500	2,340	2,220	2,160	1,880	1,740
5	5	2,940	2,560	2,400	2,260	2,200	1,920	1,780
5	6	3,000	2,620	2,460	2,320	2,250	1,950	1,810
5	7	3,070	2,680	2,520	2,380	2,310	2,000	1,850
5	8	3,140	2,740	2,580	2,440	2,370	2,060	1,900
5	9	3,200	2,800	2,640	2,500	2,430	2,100	1,930
5	10	3,280	2,880	2,710	2,560	2,490	2,160	1,990
5	11	3,360	2,950	2,790	2,620	2,550	2,210	2,040
6	0	3,440	3,030	2,860	2,680	2,610	2,250	2,070
6	1	3,520	3,130	2,940	2,740	2,670	2,310	2,130
6	2	3,600	3,180	3,010	2,800	2,730	2,370	2,180
6	3	3,680	3,250	3,090	2,860	2,790	2,410	2,220

Daily Calorie Requirement for Women of Normal Weight

Ft.	In.	15–19	20–29	30–39	40–49	50–59	60–69	70–79
4	9	2,080	1,890	1,810	1,760	1,710	1,480	1,370
4	10	2,110	1,920	1,840	1,790	1,740	1,510	1,400
4	11	2,140	1,950	1,870	1,820	1,770	1,530	1,430
5	0	2,190	1,980	1,900	1,850	1,800	1,550	1,450
5	1	2,240	2,020	1,940	1,890	1,850	1,590	1,480
5	2	2,290	2,060	1,980	1,950	1,900	1,640	1,510
5	3	2,350	2,100	2,030	2,000	1,950	1,690	1,550
5	4	2,400	2,150	2,080	2,040	2,000	1,740	1,590
5	5	2,460	2,200	2,140	2,080	2,050	1,780	1,640
5	6	2,520	2,250	2,190	2,120	2,100	1,820	1,690
5	7	2,570	2,300	2,240	2,160	2,150	1,860	1,730
5	8	2,620	2,350	2,290	2,220	2,200	1,910	1,770
5	9	2,680	2,400	2,340	2,260	2,250	1,950	1,800
5	10	2,740	2,450	2,400	2,310	2,300	1,990	1,830
5	11	2,800	2,500	2,450	2,360	2,350	2,040	1,880
6	0	2,860	2,550	2,500	2,410	2,400	2,090	1,930

* From *Clinical Nutrition* by Norman Jolliffe (New York: Harper & Row, 1972). Used with permission.

To lose a pound a week, you have to have a deficit of 3,500 calories a *week* (remember that each pound of fat equals 3,500 calories); that's 500 calories a *day*. To lose two pounds a week, you need a deficit of 7,000 calories a week; that's 1,000 calories a day. If you decide to lose a pound a week, subtract 500 calories from your present daily needs, as shown in this example:

$$
\begin{aligned}
\text{Present daily calorie needs} &= 2{,}250 \\
\text{Daily calorie deficit} &= \underline{500} \\
\text{What you should eat} &= 1{,}750 \text{ calories a day}
\end{aligned}
$$

The final figure is the amount of calories you should eat every day to lose a pound a week. You can use that as a general guide and follow your Jolliffe self-monitoring chart to find out the exact number of calories to eat a day to keep on a pound-a-week schedule. Once you start losing weight, you will find it necessary to eat somewhat less to keep your weight loss at a pound a week. That is because as you lose pounds your daily calorie needs go down.

As a handy way of keeping track of calorie counts, get yourself a calorie-count booklet from any pharmacy, dime store, or bookstore. It is small enough to carry around with you and shows the calorie count for a great many foods. If you want to go all out, you can send $1.50 to the Superintendent of Documents, U.S. Government Printing Office, Washington, D.C. 20402, and ask for *Composition of Foods*, Agriculture Handbook No. 8. This tome contains the food values of 2,483 items, from abalone to Zwieback. There is a cheaper version (twenty-five cents) called *Nutritive Value of Foods*, also available from the Superintendent of Documents. It contains only 512 items but has the advantage of including ordinary measures, like cups, scoops, slices, which makes estimating the calorie content of what you eat easier. Incidentally, when you are counting calories, don't forget to allow for the fact that most restaurant and home portions are bigger by about 25 per cent than those in most calorie-counter books. You will find that eventually you will automatically remember food values. Things will fall into categories: most meats are 300 calories, most fish 200 calories, and most vegetables 15 calories.

You can combine all three methods: restriction, menus, and counting. I appropriated that part of each plan that proved most useful to me. I had big problems with dinners, so I used the menu plan there. I restricted by cutting out ice cream, pies, and hamburgers. And I counted. Inadvertently, I discovered a behavior-control method associated with calorie-counting: I found that if I counted calories before a meal, I tended to eat less. Counting before dinner acts as part of the reward/punishment scheme. If I counted, say, 1,500 calories before sitting down to dinner, the mere thought of the number was enough to inhibit eating.

Once again, it is important to remember that your count may be off by as much as 10 per cent. So, to play safe, *add* 10 per cent to your count. If you have had 400 calories for breakfast, count it as 440; 1,000 calories for lunch goes down as 1,100. However, no matter how you count or which calorie-counting book you use, only your Jolliffe chart tells you if it is accurate. It also will reflect the difference between your calorie needs for your estimated daily activity and your actual calorie consumption in physical movement.

Remember: you need behavior-control methods to avoid in-between-meal and nighttime eating, and at those unpredictable times when you are faced with high-calorie foods. The very fact of counting calories is a deterrent to eating. You look at a piece of pie: 400 calories. But although the high number may inhibit the food response, eventually the calorie count grows weaker as punishing power unless you reinforce the deterrence.

Controlling Cholesterol

If you believe, as I do, that not only the amount but the kind of food you eat affects your health, you will want to do something about the cholesterol in your blood while you are losing weight. Fortunately, a cholesterol-lowering program goes hand in glove with a weight-reduction or weight-maintenance program. Such foods as beef, lamb, pork, and dairy products are rich in calories and also rich in the cholesterol stimulant, saturated fat.

Saturated fat? Most people have heard of polyunsaturated fat, thanks to the wide advertising campaigns of some vegetable-oil companies and to faddists who, some years ago, promoted polyunsaturated fat as the answer to dietary problems. Both terms— saturated and polyunsaturated—were invented by chemists to describe the molecular structure of fats. But many people are not aware that there are several different kinds of fat, just as there are several different kinds of sugars, proteins, and starches.

It would take several pages and a couple of diagrams to describe all these differences, and in the end I do not think that you would be in a much better position to design your diet. Accordingly, I will make a simple, although somewhat inaccurate, statement that will guide you through the morass of the chemistry of fats. It will perhaps help you untangle *saturated, mono-unsaturated* and *polyunsaturated* so that you can devise a food pattern that is the least stimulating to your body's cholesterol chemistry: The amount of saturation in a fat depends on how many hydrogen atoms a fat molecule contains; the more hydrogen, the more saturation; the less hydrogen, the less saturation, or, as a chemist would say, the more polyunsaturation.* You already know that the more saturated fat a food contains, the more it stimulates your body to produce cholesterol. The other helpful fact to remember is that the more saturated fat a mixture of fats contains, the more it tends to be solid at room temperature—a fast way of distinguishing the culprit.

Beef, lamb, pork, and milk fats, like butter and cheese, tend to be solid at room temperature; vegetable oils—corn, peanut, safflower, and olive—tend to be liquid at room temperature. Cream and coconut oil, a vegetable fat, are viscous at room temperature and highly saturated. Fish oils are liquid. Imagine a fish swimming in the cold North Atlantic with saturated fat in its tissues. It would be stiff as a board because, unlike mammals, fish have no temperature regulator; their bodies assume the temperature of the water. Thus the saturated fat would harden. Poultry fats also tend to be liquid and are less saturated than animal fats.

Mono-unsaturated fats are of intermediate saturation. Olive oil contains much mono-unsaturated fat. Vegetable oils that have

---

* For purists, the statement should more accurately read: the amount of saturation of a fat depends on what proportion of atomic positions capable of being filled by hydrogen atoms is actually filled. If all the positions are filled, the fat is said to be saturated; if only one position is unfilled, the fat is said to be mono-unsaturated; if more than one position is unfilled, the fat is said to be polyunsaturated.

been treated by hydrogenation, that is, saturated by the addition of hydrogen, are solid at room temperature. Corn-oil and safflower-oil margarines have been especially prepared so as to be solid at room temperature and yet low in saturation. As I mentioned, coconut oil is one of the few vegetable oils with high saturation. (My wife, knowing of my desire to avoid butterfat because of its high saturation, used to purchase a specially prepared "sour cream" advertised as having no butterfat. True enough. The thickening ingredient is coconut oil!)

The percentage of saturation of fats in foods varies tremendously. For example, the amount of saturated fat in lard depends on what the pig ate during his life. If he consumed large amounts of corn, his fat would be relatively unsaturated. In this respect, you could say pigs are like human beings, or vice versa. A cow's stomach (one of them at least) contains bacteria that convert unsaturated vegetable fat to saturated fat. So your steak has hard fat.

The main thing to remember is that saturated fat in your food stimulates the cholesterol-production mechanism in your body. You recall that high levels of cholesterol in your blood are associated with increased risk of atherosclerosis. Furthermore, when you eat foods containing cholesterol—all meats have some—the accompanying saturated fat facilitates the absorption of cholesterol by your body. Egg yolks, which contain both saturated fat and cholesterol in abundance, are superb cholesterol boosters. Recently, however, an artificial egg product has been made available on the market.

Examples of Fat Composition of Foods

	Saturated	*Mono-unsaturated*	*Polyunsaturated*
Beef fat	51%	47%	2%
Lard	40	49	11
Butter	61	37	2
Fish oil	16	57	37
Chicken fat	33	39	28
Corn oil	12	33	55
Coconut oil	87	9	4

Should You Drink Oil?

In the early days of cholesterol study, there were nutritionists who believed that you should actually drink vegetable oils—preferably corn or safflower—to counteract saturated fat. This is now known to be partially wrong. While polyunsaturated fat does in a sense "balance" the saturated fat, the latter is more powerful in stimulating cholesterol formation in your body than the polyunsaturates are in reducing it. If you get too much saturated fat, you cannot completely balance it with polyunsaturated fat.

The general idea is to reduce or eliminate fats—especially saturated fats—from your diet; in that way you will keep both your weight and your cholesterol level under control. Just substituting fish and poultry for beef, lamb, and pork in most meals goes a long way toward achieving that control. By drinking oil, you might increase not only the proportion of polyunsaturated fat, but the total amount of such fat. It is certainly not a natural way to take in oil (no population is known to drink oil), and it could be harmful. The more prudent course is to fashion an eating style after that of a population that has a low heart-attack rate (the Japanese, Chinese, or Italian). Keep in mind, however, that all studies show that Japanese *in Japan* and the Italians *in Italy* have a lower heart-attack rate and lower cholesterol levels than those same ethnic groups living in the United States.

The Prudent Diet

One of the first attempts to alter the average diet style was made in the 1950's by Dr. Norman Jolliffe at the New York City Department of Health. Out of that experiment arose what he called the "Prudent Diet," prudent simply because it was nutritionally sound—except for one thing. Dr. Jolliffe had his subjects drink corn oil. Even so, follow-up studies on those subjects showed that they had a lower heart-attack rate than subjects who did not follow the Prudent Diet. The studies also revealed that the Prudent Dieters lowered their blood cholesterol by an average of 12 per cent.

The pattern of eating is designed to keep the daily consumption of saturated fat *and* cholesterol below certain numerical limits. Using various food tables you could count saturated-fat and cholesterol units, just as you count calories, but that rather demanding task is not necessary, as you will see if you follow the Prudent Diet guidelines in retraining your eating habit. At the same time you can reduce the *amount* of food you eat by selecting one of the three calorie-reduction methods. Here are the guidelines:

1. *Use fish or seafood in from five to seven meals a week.* Take it easy with shrimp, lobster, clams, and oysters; they contain as much cholesterol as beef, and sometimes more. However, they are quite low in fat. Emphasize fish and you are not only substituting a low-saturated-fat and low-cholesterol food for the high-fat beef, lamb, and pork meals; you are also reducing your calorie intake by half.

Worried about mercury? The overwhelming preponderance of fish brought to market is safe. Even swordfish, considered the most dangerous, can be eaten once in a while. The risk of mercury poisoning is almost nonexistent—especially when compared with that of heart attack.

If your problem is that you cannot stand fish, give serious thought to the behavior-control methods of learning to like it that were discussed previously.

2. *Use chicken, turkey, or veal in four meals a week.* Like fish and seafood, these three are low in fat, especially the fowl. At this point you have eliminated saturated-fat meats from ten of the fourteen major meals of the week, that is, lunches and dinners.

3. *Use lean cuts of beef, pork, or lamb (if you must) for no more than three meals a week.* Before cooking, trim away all the excess fat. Broil when possible, allowing the fats to drip away. No gravies! If you like stew, let it stand overnight in the refrigerator and then skim off the congealed fat. The stew will not only be less fatty; it will taste better because the spices will have had a chance to seep into the meat and vegetables.

4. *Eat no more than four to seven eggs a week.* This is a hard blow to those who ritualistically eat two or more fried eggs for breakfast every day (not to mention uncounted hidden eggs in cakes and pastries). Two eggs contain twice the daily cholesterol limit for the average man.

5. *Use only cottage cheese or skim-milk cheese.* Cottage cheese is great in any reducing or low-fat diet. It contains practically no fat and is very rich in protein. Unfortunately, you will probably have to develop a taste for cottage cheese; it tends to be bland. But there are many recipes* in which cottage cheese can be used to great advantage. (I'm crazy about it mixed with noodles, margarine, pepper and salt, and dusted with a little Parmesan cheese.) Other cheeses are a problem because they are so tasty. No manufacturer has yet made a good, low-fat, hard cheese. Sylvia Rosenthal, whose cookbook I swear by, reports there is a Swiss import called Sapsago, made of skim milk and herbs, that is fine for grating. So far, I haven't found it on any dairy shelf. To get an idea of the cheese problem, look at this breakdown chart:

Composition of 3.5 Ounces of Various Cheeses

Cheese	Calories	Total Fat Calories	Saturated Fat Calories
Cottage			
Uncreamed	86	2.7	1.3
Creamed	106	38.0	19.0
Cream	374	340.0	192.0
Others: Swiss,			
blue, Camembert,			
Cheddar, American,			
Limburger, et cetera	345–398	190–290	100–145

Notice that creamed cottage cheese has over 35 extra calories of fat, half of them saturated. And it is getting more and more difficult to find uncreamed cottage cheese at the dairy counter. The manufacturers know their human animals: we like that extra little bit of fat. Laws that protect the dairy industry prevent manufacturers from adding unsaturated fat to cottage cheese. But if you use uncreamed cottage cheese in recipes and add margarine or oil for the fat, you will get a tasty dish. Sylvia Rosenthal

---

* My favorite low-fat, low-saturation cookbook is *Live High on Low Fat* by Sylvia Rosenthal. The American Heart Association publishes cookery pamphlets to be had for the asking. Dr. Jolliffe's and Dr. Whyte's books also contain excellent low-fat recipes.

has a recipe for a spectacularly good cheesecake made this way.

Remember: cheeses are not forbidden. Just don't eat them frequently. When you do, use them grated, as flavoring agents rather than chewable food.

6. *Lay off commercial pastries and cakes.* All of them contain lots of fat. Some bakeries use butter and are proud of it; others include hydrogenated fat (artificially saturated). The midafternoon coffee break that includes a Danish pastry or a doughnut also includes a "healthy" splash of cholesterol and saturated fat. If you can get some home-baked cookies, cakes, or pastries made with unsaturated fat and egg whites (instead of whole eggs) you can indulge—according to the limits dictated by what you are trying to achieve in calorie reduction.

You can readily see that behavior-control methods are necessary in controlling your food pattern long enough so that it becomes habitual. There are many foods that have no place in a program designed to lower blood cholesterol. At this writing, the Food and Drug Administration is moving to require manufacturers to list the fat content by source, that is, animal or vegetable, and saturation. That will be a great deal of help; but you must still be careful to avoid the high-fat foods that appear in magazine, newspaper, and television advertisements, on market shelves, and in restaurants. Only behavior control, backed by nutritional knowledge, will enable you to avoid them consistently.

Variety

So far, I have been talking about weight reduction and cholesterol control. What about nutrition in general?

You must maintain resistance to infection, and there is evidence that good nutrition increases such resistance. Vitamins help you avoid deficiency diseases; protein replaces the protein your body uses in its daily functions. Healthy blood requires iron; calcium and other elements give you healthy bones.

Much has been written about these subjects. Allow me to simplify it all with one word: variety. If you eat many different kinds of foods within the guidelines of the Prudent Diet and within your calorie needs, you will fulfill *all* your nutritional requirements. I know this is a broad statement, and I will probably get many arguments against it. But my reading of the data suggests that variety is the key.

To help you cut a trail through the vast possibilities of selection, I suggest you refer first to the sample menus previously mentioned. Notice that each meal contains foods from different categories: breads and cereals; proteins; fruits; vegetables. Select one food from each category with at least three ounces from a protein source for each meal. (You can compensate a low-protein breakfast with increased amounts at lunch and dinner.) The following list will give you some idea of the possibilities.

FRUITS. Especially the citrus fruits, but not excluding apples, grapes, pears, cantaloupe, berries, peaches, watermelon. A cup of fresh orange juice gives you the minimum amount of vitamin C advocated for adults each day. Do not rely on orange juice alone; use whole oranges and the other fruits.

BREADS. Notice the plural. If you eat only white bread made of unenriched flour, all you are getting is calories. Look for vitamin-enriched bread. Better still, look for whole-wheat bread that has much of the vitamin content left in. Again, eat a variety of different breads, leaning hard on whole wheat.

If you eat breakfast cereals, it is better to get those you have to cook, even if they are just the instant type. Steer clear of the sugar-coated cereals (especially for your children). Line up half a dozen different types that you like and then rotate through them, rather than, for example, eating cornflakes every single morning. Suggestions: oatmeal, cooked wheat, farina (enriched), wheat germ, bran and whole-wheat cereals. I include the various macaroni and spaghetti products here. If you are worried about the high calorie content, be assured that a cup of spaghetti without the sauce has the same calorie content as two and a half slices of bread . . . and a cup of spaghetti is a lot of eating. The trick is to stick to low-calorie sauce recipes.

VEGETABLES. Vegetables are terrific. They have low calorie content, are high in bulk and vitamin and mineral counts. For instance, a single carrot contains all the vitamin A you need each day (remember that other foods contain the vitamin, too). Even more important, vegetables have a wide variety of flavors, a big bonus if you are at all interested in food. Today at frozen-food counters you can get a selection of a dozen or more vegetables, which, by and large, have the same vitamin content and food value as they did the day they were picked. Indeed, they may have more value than fresh vegetables, which often spend inordinate amounts of time traveling on trains and trucks. Watch out for those frozen packages of prepared vegetable recipes; they have butter or some other saturated fat. Think of the variety: asparagus, beans, bean sprouts, beets, broccoli (another high-vitamin-A vegetable), cabbage, carrots, cauliflower, celery, collards, cucumbers, endive, lettuce, okra, peas, onions, radishes, squash, tomatoes, and on and on and on. You could have a different vegetable at every dinner for two weeks without repeating. Yet so many people settle for carrots and peas, or none. Note: do not overcook vegetables—two to seven minutes will do for most. Leave the vegetable chewy, not soggy. Treat potatoes like macaroni products. They have more vitamin C than spaghetti but that's about all. Adding cream and butter to potatoes or frying them adds calories like mad. Sweet potatoes, although rich calorically, are loaded with vitamin A and calcium.

PROTEIN SOURCES. Fish, fowl, cottage cheese, dried beans, pork, beef, and lamb. Follow the Prudent Diet guidelines—and check calorie content, too. Remember that pork has the highest caloric value per pound. Does the inclusion of beans surprise you? They have as much protein as bacon per ounce, and only a fraction of the calories. Calorie for calorie, dried beans (cooked without added fat) have more protein than a good sirloin steak. You would have to eat eleven ounces of beans (a lot) to get the same protein as four ounces of steak, but you would end up with fewer calories and no saturated fat. Unfortunately, commercially canned baked beans—except vegetarian style—have a lot of pork fat. Before you buy, check the ingredients. Remember the average-size person has to have about nine ounces a day of protein food (count four ounces of beans as two ounces). The menu plans previously discussed provide the proper amount of protein.

BEVERAGES. Most nutritionists recommend two cups of skim milk a day for adults for the calcium and protein it contains. I try to get mine from buttermilk or yogurt, both of which I prefer to skim milk. For people reared on whole milk who cannot stand the lack of creaminess in skim milk, I suggest adding skim-milk powder to regular skim milk. It increases the calories somewhat but makes a more palatable drink. Coffee, tea, and cocoa are okay unless you add cream (fresh or artificial) or whole milk. Artificial creams often contain coconut oil. Diet sodas are okay, too. Some nutritionists are very much against them, because they are empty foods. And some people have a nagging worry about "all those chemicals." My feeling is that if you need to drink something with a meal or in between meals, it is better to have a diet drink than a sugar-laden cola or other soft drink.

Wine? Why not, if taken with the meal and with the understanding that each four-ounce glass of table wine contains about 100 calories (as does eight ounces of beer), which turns out to be exactly the amount in a cola drink. But wine and beer contain fractional amounts of vitamins and minerals; soft drinks contain nothing beyond flavoring and sugar.

By this time one word should have suggested itself to you: *variety.* Select many different breads, fruits, vegetables, and protein sources. Variety is the key to getting adequate amounts of vitamins and minerals; it makes up for the food values lost through processing, improper storage, or overcooking. Recently, scientists have become concerned over the possibility that we may be deprived of certain trace metals, like zinc and magnesium, that our bodies require in minuscule amounts. Food grown in soil that is deficient in a trace metal is itself then deficient. Again, variety to the rescue. If your food comes from many different places, the insufficiencies of one soil area will be balanced out by the richness of another. The same reasoning applies if you are worried about additives and pesticides. For example, suppose some farmers in one part of your state erred in dusting their potatoes with too much of a particular chemical. If you eat potatoes day after day and they happen to come from that region, you will load up on that chemical. But if you have potatoes one day, rice another, spaghetti a third, the chances of eating rice, wheat, and potatoes grown by farmers who all made the same mistake in the same season is low. Probably all farmers use chemicals; I'm not excusing that. I am saying that variety insures against your getting a bigger dose than you might get by eating few foods.

Organic foods have been touted as being more "healthful" because they are grown without chemicals. Aside from the difficulty of determining whether the food you are buying is really organically grown, there is little, if any, scientific evidence that organic foods prevent disease or increase life expectancy.

Avoidances

One does not talk about prohibitions; "avoidances" suggests minimal use. Besides, eating in restaurants makes it almost impossible to eliminate many items; butter is one. I have already mentioned many foods to avoid; the following grouping will make it easier to remember.

BAKED GOODS. Cakes, pies, pastries, cookies, doughnuts, muffins, waffles, sweet rolls . . . all contain heavy loads of hydrogenated fat, butter, or eggs, or all three. Many also contain chocolate, another saturated vegetable fat. And the calorie content of such baked goods is correspondingly sky high, not only from fat but also from sugar. A slice of pie has more calories than a small steak. Try baking at home, using recipes that call for egg white and unsaturated vegetable oil. You can make baked goods that will adhere to the calorie or food-intake limits you have set for yourself. If you use enriched flour, you can sometimes substitute some baked sweet thing for bread, on a calorie basis. There are two exceptions to the ban on commercial baked goods: angel food cake is made from egg whites and practically no fat. Sponge cake runs a close second. Nix on cheesecake unless it is made at home with cottage cheese.

DAIRY PRODUCTS. Butter, cheese (except cottage), cream, ice cream, ice milk (but if you *must* have something like ice cream, this has somewhat less fat and fewer calories than ice cream), whole milk, custard (unless made at home with skim milk and egg white) and other puddings. You can use any of the corn- or safflower-oil margarines. Check labels for ingredients; stay away from those that contain coconut oil or animal fats. You do not have to buy special medicinal margarines—remember, the important thing is to reduce saturated fats, not raise unsaturated fats. Use hard cheeses only as flavoring, not as food.

PREPARED MEAT PRODUCTS. Hot dogs, baloney, liverwurst, salami, corned beef, pastrami, head cheese—all contain prodigious amounts of animal fat. Some have fat added to them over and above the natural fat content of the meat. Until manufacturers produce low-fat prepared-meat products properly labeled, I would stay away from them.

DESSERTS. Ice cream, baked goods, candies, especially chocolate, contain either animal or saturated-vegetable fats. Instead, choose fruits, nuts, nut candies, seed candies, jelly beans or gum drops, gelatin desserts and home-created desserts with low fat content. Keep in mind that except for fruits, most desserts exact a high caloric toll.

ALCOHOL. Dr. Jolliffe devised a quick way of checking caloric values of alcoholic drinks: multiply 1 calorie by the proof of the liquor and that by the number of ounces (of course it doesn't include the sugar you add). Thus two ounces of 90-proof whisky contains 180 calories, or the equivalent of two and a half slices of non-vitamin-enriched bread. Dr. Jolliffe called alcohol calories "empty calories." If you add sugar or a soft drink, a single mixed drink costs you 205 calories; two drinks, 410 calories—or the equivalent of a six-ounce steak. Sixteen ounces of beer also has 200 calories, as does eight ounces of wine. It is probably a good idea to limit your alcohol intake to under 400 calories a day, preferably to 200. This limitation is based not only on calorie control, but on the potential risk of alcohol habituation.

SALT. Surprised? You shouldn't be. Although salt is an essential nutrient, too much may induce high blood pressure. Studies indicate that individuals who salt food before tasting it have higher blood pressure than those who don't salt before they taste. A good rule is: taste first, then salt—and use less than you have been. (Use behavior-control techniques.) The Japanese have low cholesterol rates, but they have somewhat higher stroke rates than Americans. It has been suggested that the reason is that their food is saltier, which leads to high blood pressure. My only rule about salt is not to salt at all unless I feel that the food would be impossible to eat without it.

SUGAR. Many foods, particularly fruit and vegetables, contain sugars of various kinds; the sugar in milk is lactose. However, in the past one hundred years, Western man has increased his consumption of refined sugar enormously—threefold in less than a century. Refined sugar—granulated and confectioners'—was practically unknown in medieval times. For people with diabetes—a condition in which the body cannot handle sugar—the chance of having atherosclerosis is relatively high. Nobody yet knows whether if sugar intake is reduced the risk of atherosclerosis is also. But it is known that reducing sugar intake softens the symptoms of diabetes.

There are evidently millions of individuals whose body chemistry is stimulated by the intake of sugar to produce fats called "triglycerides"—a process analogous to the stimulation of cholesterol production by fats. There is some evidence suggesting that just as your risk of atherosclerosis goes up with high levels of blood cholesterol, it also goes up with high levels of blood triglycerides. Some theorists think that sugar alone stimulates the body to create triglycerides; others are of the opinion that carbohydrates (starches *and* sugars) stimulate the triglyceride chemistry. Starches are contained in bread, rice, macaroni, potatoes. Sugar is a simple carbohydrate; starches a complex carbohydrate. There is data to indicate that alcohol also triggers triglyceride production. There is a growing feeling that if you do eat carbohydrates, you should eat them as starches rather than sugars. Starches seem to stimulate the triglyceride mechanism to a lesser degree.

If you follow the Prudent Diet and the meal patterns suggested, and avoid the foods in this section, you will dramatically reduce your refined-sugar intake. Because you will be keeping your weight low, you will automatically reduce your carbohydrate intake to the minimum required by your body. You may be increasing the *proportion* of carbohydrates as you drop fat from your foods, but not the *quantity*. Forget about the low-carbohydrate diet, also called the Drinking Man's Diet. Nutritionally, it is nonsense.

One more point: in recent years scientists have discovered that certain individuals are peculiarly sugar sensitive, that is, they produce an excessive amount of triglycerides after eating sugar and, to some extent, starch, and after drinking alcohol. Tests to determine whether you are one of these individuals can be done at present only by a few laboratories, and only a few physicians know how to interpret them. But eventually such individuals, along with those who are fat sensitive, will benefit from scientific progress. Then it will be possible to design food patterns for each type that will provide optimum protection against atherosclerosis and other diseases. In the meantime, the Prudent Diet, coupled with a food intake designed to keep your weight optimal, gives you the greatest chance of lowering your risk, whether or not you are one of these types.

Vitamins

Should you take vitamin pills? A hard question. Many nutritionists say that varied diet (precisely the kind I am urging you to adopt) will provide all the vitamins a healthy person needs. Make no mistake, you need vitamins daily to carry out the body chemistry of growth and repair. But, except for vitamin D, which your skin produces if you spend time in the sun, your body cannot create vitamins. So you must get them from either food or pills.

Unfortunately, most Americans do not eat a varied diet of the kind I have been discussing. Monotonous eaters should probably take some sort of multiple-vitamin pill daily. However, it must be remembered that vitamin pills alone do not cause the really vital changes: reduction of animal fat, reduced total fat, reduced sugar, reduced calorie intake.

Some doctors prescribe high-dose vitamins in the case of certain diseases, for pregnant women, for old people, and for infants. They know that the average person has not really learned to vary his diet sufficiently to counteract a specific vitamin drain. In infants, the diet is so monotonous that the likelihood of vitamin deficiency is high. In the case of certain diseases, the vitamin requirement is enormously high, doses that could not be provided by any available food.

Dr. Linus Pauling, a chemist who has won two Nobel prizes, has started a controversy by urging large amounts of vitamin C as a preventative for colds or to abort infection if a cold has already started. Dr. Pauling found evidence in human experiments to support his thesis. But the treatment needs to be tested on a much larger scale, with scrupulous attention to possible bad side effects, before vitamin C in large doses can be recommended as an acceptable preventative.

The amount of vitamin C required by Dr. Pauling's anticold treatment is equivalent to that found in two and a half quarts of orange juice a day. That would also give you 1,000 calories. So pills would seem to be the only way out—but I would not take them, at least not at the present time.

You now have all the information you need about food and habits to change your daily eating pattern. The steps are easy: decide which pattern you want to adopt for low weight and low blood cholesterol; then apply behavior-control and food-intake methods to achieve that pattern.

One warning: human beings are contrary animals. While they often respond to reward and punishment as easily as a pigeon, their ability to rationalize sometimes defeats their will. They may with one part of their mind want to lose weight and control food; but another part rationalizes away the need to do either. That rationalization may be imbedded in an emotional state that has been thoroughly reinforced by the anxiety relief derived from eating patterns.

What I am saying finally is that the methods in this book are not sure-fire; they give you only a fighting chance to win a war with yourself, for yourself.

8 / So You Don't Use Drugs

The Drug Society

Since nearly 100 per cent of the American adult population uses drugs in some form, ours must be labeled a drug society. If you think you're exempt from membership, consider the following.

First, the definition: a drug is any substance, other than food, that, when consumed, alters the functioning of the body. Chemicals that reduce pain, make you sleep, kill germs inside your body, lower blood pressure, stimulate your brain or heart, or both, are all drugs. Some perform only one function, but almost all affect many parts of the body. And few drugs have no unwanted side effects.

When a doctor prescribes drugs, we tend to think of them as medicine. But millions of people take drugs without a doctor's prescription. They swallow aspirin, cough syrups, cold pills, sleep tablets, laxatives, stay-awake pills, and antacids, just to mention a few kinds of the estimated 250,000 products you can buy over the counter without a slip of paper from a physician.

Recently, the word drugs has come to have a special, pejorative meaning. When people speak of the "drug problem," they usually mean mood-changing chemicals, particularly drugs like heroin, cocaine, and morphine. The drug idea usually also includes a large variety of other, milder mood-changing substances: marijuana, amphetamines, barbiturates, LSD, mescaline, and tranquilizers; all are being taken regularly by millions of people in both legal and illegal ways.

If you still feel that you have nothing to do with drugs because you take none of the above chemicals, consider the fact that there are mood-changing substances in cigarettes, coffee, tea, and cocoa. Cigarettes contain nicotine, a powerful stimulant. Coffee and tea contain caffeine, also a stimulant, and cocoa has a chemical cousin of caffeine. None of these can be classified as a food, because without cream and sugar they, like cigarettes, have a food value of zero.

Finally, there is the most dangerous drug in America: alcohol, the mood-changing drug par excellence. Indeed, if alcohol were not centuries old and thoroughly entrenched in our social mores, the Food and Drug Administration would probably make it available by prescription only.

If you partake of none of the drugs mentioned above, not even an aspirin or a cup of tea, then, indeed, you can count yourself out of the drug society. But if you pop any kind of pill, with or without prescription, or puff a cigarette, sip a drink—alcohol, coffee, tea—you have a decision to make. You must first learn about the risk to your mind and body. No drug is without risk, in either the short or long run, although, of course, some drugs, like heroin and alcohol, carry greater risk than others, like aspirin and tea. For still others, like marijuana, the risk is unknown. But with *all* drugs you must decide if the risks are worth the immediate benefits.

A physician makes a similar judgment when he writes a prescription. He knows that no drug is completely safe; in fact, if a chemical is not in some way harmful, it is probably completely ineffective as medicine. An effective drug must produce bodily changes, and for some people the changes are undesirable. Aspirin, for example, causes stomach bleeding in a considerable number of individuals, and in some even hemorrhaging. Thus, a physician will warn ulcer patients about using aspirin. On the other hand, in dealing with a cancer patient, he will suggest the most dangerous substances—some that bring the patient to the outer edge of life—in an effort to stem the disease.

It is the familiar problem of estimating risk versus benefit. Unfortunately, too often we do not or cannot face that problem, consciously or rationally. Those of us who have formed habits with certain drugs tend to underestimate the risk and overestimate the benefits. Furthermore, since the harm we suffer usually lies at some remote time and the pleasure potential is imminent, our decision at any moment is heavily weighted for use of a drug. Even when its harmfulness has been established incontrovertibly, we still tend to make exceptions of ourselves, as in the case of cigarettes, for instance.

The habitual taking of drugs—the morning coffee, the drink at lunchtime, the cigarette, the pep pill—also makes any action on a rational risk-versus-benefit basis extremely difficult. The time to make a decision is before habits are formed. But even that may be difficult. In our social environment drug-taking appears to be as natural as eating. Almost all of us have been urged by friends at one time or another to take aspirin, to have a drink, to smoke a cigarette, to sip some coffee or tea; and today increasing numbers of us have been offered marijuana, LSD, heroin, cocaine, and other drugs that are not legal. Such offers are hard to turn down, so strong is our gregarious nature.

Getting into Drugs

By now you know enough about the principles of reinforcement in habit formation to understand how many people get so involved with drugs that they cannot let go. These principles are gaining ascendancy as the major theory of addiction to drugs like heroin and cocaine. But what are the major reinforcement factors?

The drug taker—the cigarette smoker, alcohol drinker, tea sipper—is usually part of a social milieu in which the taking of a particular drug is common and approved. He may be born into that environment, as the Irish are born into a drinking culture. Or, for a new experience, he may seek out a society or group where drug-taking is common. Experience-seeking is not necessarily related to drugs, however. Among the young, experimentation is as old as civilization. It has created a constant disturbance in society as, generation after generation, young people—particularly bright young people—attempted to break with the mores of their elders. With each generation, the fashion changes. For some it has been social revolution, for others religious innovation; more recently it is sex and drugs, although neither of these was unknown in past generations.

The creation of a particular fashion is not a well-understood phenomenon. We know that styles in clothing can be relatively easily manipulated by the trendsetters of Paris and New York. And something like that may happen in behavior. The role of men like Dr. Timothy Leary, the apostle of LSD, in setting a trend among young intellectuals should not at all be underestimated. For a time, Leary, a Harvard professor, seemed to have projected the authority in drug fashion of a Dior in clothes.

An easy and popular generalization about drug-taking behavior is that it is a symptom of a "sick" society, a society that was until recently involved in an immoral war in Southeast Asia, is too affluent and materialistic while at the same time grinding down its minorities, particularly the blacks. In the absence of data, of course, any sort of theory seems plausible; for some people the mere assertion of a connection between drugs and a sick society proves the case. They make an appealingly simple conclusion: if our society were not sick, there would be no drug problem.

Consider the fact that, whatever the morality of the war in Southeast Asia, there has been a world-wide increase in the use of mood-changing drugs even in countries that were not involved in the war. England is an example. In my opinion, the war, for the theory to be plausible, should be a basic factor in most cases of increased national drug use. It is not.

Affluence must be considered as a possible factor. Young people today do have more spending money than in the past, and undoubtedly some of that money goes to buy mood-changing drugs—cigarettes, alcohol, pep pills, and the rest. But it is also true that poverty-stricken young people in the ghettos of America use mood-changing drugs heavily, more heavily than do young people of the middle class, with the possible exception of marijuana, which is becoming a middle-class drug. There have been generations in which poor people used drugs and others in which they did not; there have been affluent times in which drug use was widespread among the middle class (laudanum, or tincture of opium, among well-off Englishwomen of Victorian times is one example), and there have been times when the middle class eschewed all drugs. Thus the presence or absence of affluence is interesting just because it is *not* a conclusive factor in drug use.

If I may guess, with some data in my corner, there are three kinds of social groups in which drug use or nonuse may be explicable:

The first is strongly fundamentalist in religion, tending to avoid drugs—alcohol, pills, et cetera. In the United States, for example, Bible-Belt Baptists use little alcohol or other mood-changing chemicals.

In the second type of social group the pervading spirit is Apollonian—in which moderation, rationality, and meditation are fundamental values. This group seems to avoid heavy dependence on drugs, although they do use them. Old-World Jews and Italians fit this description; second- and third-generation Jews in this country, less so.

The value system in the third social group is Dionysian—that is, where having a good time, pleasure-seeking, avoidance of discomfort are central. This group seems to lean toward heavy drug use. Young black males, Latins, and Irish seem to fit this category. Heavy use of alcohol is almost completely explicable by reference to the social environment. Similarly, in the 1950's, '60's, and '70's the world has seen a generation grow up in which having a good time replaced older values of duty, striving for achievement, and generational respect. When the fashion for having a good time (sometimes translated as having a transcendental experience) happens to be drug related, the explosion of chemical experiences should not be surprising.

And again the question is: What forms the fashion? To what degree is it generated by the Timothy Learys, the Allen Ginsbergs, the Beatles? Or are they all merely echoes of a movement in fashion already well under way? Without hard scientific evidence, it is almost useless to speculate; it may even be harmful, because it diverts attention from a more central concept in drug-habit formation, a concept that can have immediate practical application for the individual who wishes to avoid or break a habit.

The Reinforcement Idea

If you find yourself in a social group in which drug-taking is common and approved, the chances are that you will try the drug of fashion that is offered to you—cigarettes, alcohol, pot, et cetera. Accordingly, close to 100 per cent of Americans have tried at least one cigarette and 85 per cent have had at least one drink of alcohol. Of course, one drink or smoke does not make a habitual user (just as one shot of morphine does not create a morphine addict—although I do not advocate even one).

To form a drug habit, you must use the drug repeatedly and obtain some reward for doing so. At first, the reward is social—approval by one's peers or self-approval for having undertaken a popularly accepted or adult activity. For a boy, puffing a cigarette or taking a drink may be governed as much by the insistence of his friends as by his own manly view of himself; for girls, smoking provides a self-image of sophistication or sexiness. Those social rewards and supports must be fairly powerful, because the first few trials with almost any drug produce physical effects that are downright uncomfortable. Cigarettes produce coughing and choking; cigars, nausea; alcohol, stomach upset and dizziness; heroin, overwhelming fear and nausea; LSD, terror. Marijuana, for many people, creates no physical or mental effect the first time, making it easy for social reinforcement to cause continuation of its use.

As the drug experimenter repeats his experience, his body begins to tolerate the adverse effects. Out of the multiple responses of mind and body he learns to distinguish the pleasurable from the unpleasurable. With some drugs, the distinctions are made more rapidly than for others. Drugs like heroin, morphine, and cocaine are powerfully rewarding; others, like cigarettes, coffee, and tea, less so.

At the beginning of this period, the drug user is in a position to form a drug habit. As he takes the drug, he is immediately rewarded by the pleasure response: the lift of the cigarette inhalation; the calming effect of alcohol; the sexual throb of heroin injection; the delusions and illusions generated by LSD; the dream state created by marijuana; the intense stimulation of cocaine.

Of course, the more frequently the drug is taken, the more strongly the habit is confirmed. Take cigarettes as an example. The average smoker takes ten puffs on a single cigarette before he uses it up. Each inhalation is rewarded by the lift effect of nicotine and the taste of the tars. A smoker who takes in two packs a day puffs and is rewarded 400 times a day, or about 150,000 times a year! Even if the cigarette reward is mild, 150,000 reinforcements a year is enough to make any habit rock-firm.

Remember, too, that the more immediate the reinforcement the more powerful it is in confirming behavior. With cigarettes and with most other drugs, the reward follows within seconds after the drug is taken.

Each drug has its own reinforcing power. and the more powerful the reward, the fewer the trials needed for habitualization. Although, for most people, heroin, morphine, and cocaine do not require many trials to create a habit, they do not induce habit formation after one or even a few trials.

Addiction, Habit, Dependency

There has been much confusion over the concepts of addiction, habit, and dependency. Even drug experts have problems with clear definitions. To me, the words are interchangeable because they simply describe repetitious behavior in the presence of a signal for starting that behavior. Somebody lights a cigarette near a smoker and that signals the train of behavior to start smoking. A heroin addict is offered some heroin and he takes it. The strength of the habit, addiction, or dependency depends on how often the person involved responds to the stimulus when it is presented. A man who cannot refuse a drink has a strong drinking habit. Another who drinks regularly but can easily refuse a drink has a weaker drinking habit.

The confusion arises when for some people there seems to be no external signal for the start of the drug-taking behavior. The person merely reports a craving for the drug. In such cases, the drug-taking has been so prolonged that the slightest external signal or internal bodily change can trigger the train of activity for seeking the drug. Some drugs—heroin, alcohol, and barbiturates—produce profound bodily changes; withdrawal of the drugs creates physical symptoms, among them nausea, trembling, and chills. The onset of such changes, or even the presumed onset, is enough to signal the start of drug-taking for people who have used these drugs a long time.

When one observes a person who has been termed an addict

one sees an individual who returns again and again to his drug. If you take it away, he seeks it out. There is nothing different in this from the behavior of a person with a "drug habit" or a person who is "dependent" on a drug. It is the behavior that counts. The greater his addiction, habit, or dependency—pick your own word—the more persistently does he return to the drug, even in the face of increasing psychological, social, and physical punishment or threat of punishment.

Many people believe that physical dependency is the only sign of addiction; that is, they believe only drugs like heroin are truly addicting because upon withdrawal there are physical symptoms. However, amphetamines and cocaine, for which there are no *physical* symptoms when the drug is removed, create the same sort of strong habit that heroin can. Indeed, some believe that cocaine is far more addicting than heroin because for many the rewarding nature of the stimulation is more powerful in inducing repetition of the drug-taking behavior.

Physical dependency on drugs like heroin, morphine, alcohol, and barbiturates is real enough, however. But the theory of reinforcement suggests that it is only a negative reinforcement of an already established habit.

For example, imagine a rat in a cage in which there is a pedal bar that the animal has learned to press with its paw. At various intervals of time a bell rings and within five seconds after the ring an electric shock is delivered to the rat's feet unless he presses the bar. After a few experiences with the bell and the shock, the rat will press the bar every time the bell rings.

In the case of addiction, the "bell" is the first vague sense of discomfort that the addict feels when he has not had his drug for a few hours or days. The electric shock is analogous to the nausea, the trembling, the delirium he will feel if he continues to withhold the drug. To avoid the shock of these withdrawal symptoms, the addict takes the drug. Heroin addicts say they take heroin to "feel normal." However, the origin of the habit and whether or not to continue it depend more on the rewarding features of the drug than on the anticipated punishment that accompanies withdrawal.

One of the more persistent theories of addiction holds that a drug creates a biochemical change in the body that, in turn, produces the irresistible desire for it. In the case of alcohol, where the chemical problem has been most studied, the search for such a change has proved vain, although there are physical changes that occur over a long period of time. One is tolerance: drug users find that they must increase their drug intake with time in order to maintain the level of rewarding effects. After a period of tolerance, long-time alcohol drinkers find that less alcohol will produce the desired effects—but that's only because the liver has become inefficient in destroying the alcohol, allowing more of it to stay in the blood and reach the brain.

Another, quite popular theory asserts that addiction results from a particular personality deficit. But so far the search for the alcoholic personality or the heroin-addict personality has been in vain. In part the difficulty stems from the fact that psychologists and psychiatrists can at best only speculate about the addict's preaddictive personality and life style, both of which have been dramatically changed by his drug-seeking behavior. The heroin addict, for example, is usually described as weak, immature, and psychologically dependent. But was he that way before he started using heroin? Some drug experts say yes, but they have little evidence to back up their contention.

The sequence of events for drug-habit (addiction) formation for any drug seems to be as follows:

1. The potential drug user finds himself in a social milieu where the use of a particular drug or a number of drugs is common and approved. It is in fashion.

2. Social encouragement from friends or self-encouragement (for social reasons) leads to a few trials of the drug. At first it may produce uncomfortable effects, but these are overridden by the stronger reinforcement of self- or social approval.

3. The drug user becomes increasingly aware of its pleasurable effects, which may be tranquilizing, stimulating, delusion-creating, sedative, or just diverting.

4. The pleasurable effects can then become the reinforcing agent for the act of taking the drug. The more pleasurable the effects, the more powerful the reinforcement, and the more likely it is that the drug will become a habit or addiction.

5. Those drugs that produce physical dependence, like heroin, morphine, alcohol, and barbiturates (and, some say, cigarettes),

negatively reinforce the habit and prevent easy exit. Powerful reinforcing drugs like cocaine and amphetamines can induce strong habits without physical dependence; that is, they may be addictive.

The Drug Personality

It cannot be emphasized sufficiently that mere drug use does not inevitably lead to addiction. It may come as a surprise to many that there are heroin *users* who are not addicted, who stop taking the drug almost at will for long periods of time. However, because of the powerful habit-forming character of heroin, such individuals are rare. Similarly, it is a common observation that there are millions of alcohol *users* who are not addicted. Nor is it true that occasional barbiturate or amphetamine use always leads to addiction. But there is risk.

I would not, for example, suggest that each person try heroin as part of his life experience (though, alas, it is fashionable in some circles to suggest that everybody try everything). At present, since there are no available data on the personality characteristics that make a person particularly predisposed to drug-taking, there is no way of telling in advance who will be addicted and who will not. It has been discovered that there are individuals for whom the effects of drugs carry a particularly strong reinforcement; they learn to use drugs to change their moods from bad to good. These are the people who run the greatest risk of becoming addicts. Unfortunately, many young people have the attitude of the soldier on the battlefield: the bullet is meant for somebody else. The heroin experimenter often believes that he will be able to quit any time.

Who Needs Them?

Someone who has even moderately informed himself about drugs must rationally conclude that each one carries its own risk of addiction, its own consequences in health and disability, and its own financial and legal burdens. Against all this, one weighs the potential benefits, if any. But the common conception about drugs is that they are something that changes your mood, gives you a "feeling," or affects your brain or senses. For millions of people today it is the fashion to take such drugs as nicotine, alcohol, marijuana, LSD, cocaine, and pep pills for "fun," "experience," "relaxation," and "getting high."

I cannot give you the data on the mood changers without first giving you my position on them. It is an ancient, Apollonian cry of moderation: Who needs them? I find the world so interesting, so exciting, so much fun, and so enthralling that I do not need to even consider turning to drugs. Why start a fireworks display in my brain when there is so much going on there already?

But even if some or all of the above were not true, I would still have a negative reaction to drugs. That is because I have spent a quarter of a century observing the world of medicine, in which doctors give drugs with benefit in mind but often generate more disaster instead. There is a name for drug-induced catastrophe: iatrogenic disease (Greek for "treatment generating"). One doctor I know, who is in charge of a ward in a great New York institution, estimates that half the patients in his care are there with iatrogenic complications. Iatrogenic disease is the most rapidly rising affliction in America. And it is being produced by the very men and women—doctors—who supposedly know the most about drugs.

Thus I am wary even of taking so much as an aspirin for a headache. And I know that even the best-studied compounds are only partially understood. Scientists are just now beginning to unravel the mystery of how aspirin works. For all but a few chemicals—nicotine and alcohol among the exceptions—practically nothing is known about the short- or long-term effects on the human body.

If you take a drug for nonmedical reasons, you can estimate the value of the experience for yourself. But it is impossible to know the risks, much less how to reduce them. A skillful, conscientious doctor who prescribes a drug watches for bad side effects; when he sees them, he either stops the medicine altogether, changes it, or reduces the dosage. But the amateur is simply without the knowledge or the will to take such steps.

Yet, despite remonstrations to the contrary, people continue to take drugs for nonmedical reasons, particularly young people, who somehow believe they are invulnerable and even immortal.

For this reason, I think it is necessary to present here the available risk data. Much of it is controversial. In compiling the material, I have attempted to stick closely to the basic scientific studies of the drugs and steer clear of opinion. Some of the findings will surprise you: for example, physically speaking, heroin appears to be safer than alcohol. But we'll come to that. First, let's look at long-term consequences.

After Twenty Years

Much of the drug information we have concerns the short-term effects. We know about marijuana and brain changes (mostly minor), and about alcohol and liver (two drinks a day can produce fatty infiltration). But nothing is known about what happens to a person's body after twenty years of taking, say, barbiturates; or if people who take mood changers die faster than those who do not, or if they end up with more diseases or particular kinds.

The chief reason for the slow accumulation of data on long-term effects of drug use lies in the fact that thousands of people must be observed for a long period of time. A comparison study of nearly two hundred thousand male smokers and nonsmokers finally established a connection between smoking and lung cancer, a disease that develops after twenty years of smoking. That same study also produced evidence that cigarettes trigger heart attacks.

The ordinary person observing his smoking and nonsmoking friends could not even imagine that the cigarette habit causes lung cancer. Suppose you have one hundred male friends whose smoking habits you know. If they are between the ages of forty-five and sixty-four, only one will die each year, probably of a heart attack. Even after five years, with five of your friends dead, what conclusion will you be able to draw about smoking and longevity? None. That is why it is sheer nonsense for pot smokers to conclude that since they and all their friends smoke and nothing has happened to them, pot must be safe. However safe marijuana may be in the short run, no smoker can make any statement based on his own experience or that of his friends about the long run.

As of 1971 something like twenty-four million people had tried marijuana; something less than a million used it regularly. There is no definite figure on barbiturates, amphetamines, LSD, and the other drugs, but it must be several million overall. Ironically, however, not enough people have been users for a long enough period; in order to study the effects, scientists would have to find two hundred thousand long-time users and then check up on them at yearly intervals for at least five years (the plan followed in the tobacco studies). Because most users take drugs illegally, the difficulty of follow-up is multiplied tenfold. Such studies would cost in the neighborhood of one million dollars each, but they might be well worth the money.

Where does that leave you? Nowhere, at least at present. If you are considering using mood-changing drugs on your own, without a doctor's supervision, the long-term risk factor is a question mark—and that doesn't mean it is zero. The prudent man or woman simply does not dive off the diving board without knowing if there is water in the pool.

The Known Risks

The real and known risks in using mood-changing drugs include damage to the organs of your body, addiction, change of personality, legal punishment, impairment of physical function, decline of sex drive, intellectual confusion, social malfunctioning, and the possibility of suicide. Too many antidrug authorities list these hazards as if all drugs generated them. Alas, this overkill has worked against drug control; it is clear to the merest drug tyro that most drug users are not experiencing these risks. Consequently, drug users and nonusers alike simply discount the voice of authority.

What follows is a compendium of drugs and the risks you run in taking them.

MARIJUANA. Marijuana seems to have become the third-leading leisuretime drug, close behind tobacco and alcohol. Mostly, the users smoke a cigarette made from the leaves of the marijuana plant—hemp—which contain a drug called tetrahydrocannabinol. But marijuana can also be eaten. As with all drugs, the effects on mood and sensation depend on the amount you take.

In its mildest form, as a cigarette, the drug induces a dreamy state in which sounds, lights, and time are somewhat distorted. As most Americans use it, the dose is so low that the first-time smoker feels nothing at all. Some experts claim that the effects are so marginal that you actually have to be told about them in order to recognize them. The effective chemical exists in such small amounts that a technique of smoking—a deep and held inhalation—has to be learned in order to concentrate enough of the chemical to provide the mood change.

Distortions of vision, hearing, or other perceptions are called hallucinations, and marijuana is classed as a hallucinogenic drug. The hemp-plant varieties found in the Near and Far East and the flowers and leaves of the American-grown hemp plant contain tetrahydrocannabinol in especially high concentration. This hashish, or "hash," produces the strongest distortions.

A moderate dose of marijuana usually induces a dreamy state and an accompanying lassitude. Contrary to the antimarijuana propaganda of forty years ago, the relaxed feelings do not induce criminal activity. In higher doses, marijuana can be activating, but the more sought-after effect is sensate intensification. Appreciation of music expands; geometric patterns take on new esthetic meanings; time seems to stretch—seconds into minutes, minutes into hours. There have been reports of increased sexual abilities and appreciation, caused, perhaps, by the general disinhibiting forces that are brought into play by the drug. So much for the benefits. What about the risks?

For the vast majority of users of American-style marijuana, the risks seem quite low in the short run, certainly lower than those of alcohol, and possibly lower than those of tobacco. There are some reports of transient psychological panic, usually among older, first-time users and young persons who are emotionally unstable. It should be pointed out that emotional instability often carries with it a denial of the emotional problem, and so will not be counted as a risk by the marijuana experimenter. Rarely, doctors have reported psychotic breakdowns among marijuana users, but again there were other, complicating factors that made it difficult to put the blame on marijuana alone. Many doctors feel that the adverse psychic effects appear more frequently with the higher-potency hashish.

It is not uncommon to find among the large number of individuals, particularly young people, who have taken up a life style in which marijuana plays a central role one or more of the following personality characteristics: lack of competitiveness, an unwillingness to take conventional jobs, a refusal to regard conventional mores as binding. These have been established as merely coincident with marijuana use; to try to make the drug a causal factor would be to go beyond the evidence presently available.

What, then, can we conclude from the data? Marijuana apparently does no psychic harm to those individuals who are emotionally stable and whose life style is conventional. No physical damage from moderate use of the drug, that is, once or twice a week, has been discovered. Marijuana has a low addiction potential. However, since smoking it is rewarding in some way, it can act as a reinforcer, and as such it has the power to habitualize. What the degree of the power is, compared, say, to that of ice cream, other rich foods, or tobacco, is not yet known—not enough people have been studied closely enough. (It was only in 1968, more than fifty years after Americans began smoking tobacco cigarettes heavily, that Dr. Daniel Horn and his associates were able to understand in detail the habit-forming properties of tobacco.)

That some heavy users are addicted there can be no doubt. They show the signs: persistent returning, again and again, to the drug and, when it is removed, seeking it out no matter what the effort required.

Does marijuana lead to other, harder drugs? No, according to all available evidence. The issue has been confused by studies of heroin users who all reported that they smoked marijuana before they shot heroin. But they also reported using alcohol and tobacco, as well as amphetamines and barbiturates. These facts suggest that there is a group of individuals in our society who experiment with all sorts of drugs. They constantly seek out fellow drug users for social support and, in so doing, discover additional varieties of drugs to try.

Summary: Moderate, infrequent use of marijuana (also known as "pot," "grass," and "dope") carries low psychic and physical risks. Addiction potential is present but low. Heavy use of high-concentration substances, like hashish, raises risk. Dangers of long-term use are unknown, and there is no evidence for escalation to other, more addictive drugs.

BARBITURATES. These are the most commonly used sleeping pills. They work. They put you to sleep, sometimes permanently. Because they produce sleep, barbiturates have the highest rate of *illegal* use among older Americans, that is, over thirty-five. Their effects, similar to those of alcohol, are drowsiness, foggy memory, and inarticulate speech. If you take a large dose of barbiturates, your friends will think you are drunk.

We can thank doctors for promoting the use of these drugs; for nearly seventy years too many have been handing out barbiturates indiscriminately. There is high risk of barbiturate poisoning: because the chemical dulls memory, the taker often pops too many pills and lapses into a coma. One victim in ten dies. Half of the deaths are labeled "suicide."

There does not seem to be any short-term major physical damage from moderate use of barbiturates. (As usual, the long run is a blank.) However, the addiction potential is great, perhaps as great as that of alcohol, somewhat less than that of heroin: the user has to take increased amounts to keep getting the same effect (tolerance), and he seeks out the drug when deprived of it; in addition, barbiturates produce physical dependence, not a necessary condition for addiction, but a complicating one. When the user tries to get off the pills, he suffers dizziness, cramps, sometimes convulsions, and, in some cases, rapid and rather painful death. Although there has been some success in treating heroin, morphine, and alcohol addicts, nobody knows how to treat barbiturate addicts successfully and safely. One doctor told me: "Give me a heroin addict any time over somebody stuck on barb."

Summary: Short-term physical damage seems low; psychic damage, moderate to high. Addiction potential is high, treatment doubtful or nil. The long-term risks are unknown.

STIMULANTS. Feelings of fatigue and tiredness can be overcome—temporarily—by taking any of a number of stimulating chemicals. The most common are nicotine, caffeine, cocaine, and the amphetamines. The last are products of the chemical laboratory; the first three are derived from plants. All have the property of increasing alertness. All have addiction potential.

The dangers of nicotine, in tobacco, are fully discussed elsewhere in this book. Caffeine, in my view, is habit-forming, although the potential seems to be lower than that of tobacco. Coffee and tea contain caffeine. It appears to improve mental capacities and sharpen the senses; typists, for instance, seem to work faster and with fewer errors after a cup of coffee. But caffeine can cause an increase in the number of mistakes if you are trying to learn a skill that requires delicate co-ordination. Short-term physical and psychic damage seems low. One study has established a tentative connection between coffee-drinking (but not tea-drinking) and increased risk of heart attack.

Cocaine, found in coca leaves, may be the most addictive drug known, when injected, although, surprisingly, it does not produce any *physical* symptoms on withdrawal. Habituation is rapid. Users seek it out at all costs, and they report an undiminished craving for the stimulation it provides. The craving is excessive, more than for any other drug. If the user attempts withdrawal, he finds himself in a state of extreme fatigue and mental depression. Suicide is not an unusual result.

There is no question that cocaine causes a person to work harder and longer, both physically and intellectually; he feels that he has enormous physical and mental capacities on which to draw—although in both cases he is notorious for overestimating. Feelings of aggression and of persecution also characterize the cocaine user—in fact, it was these that created the image of the "dope fiend" at the turn of the century. Thus, psychic damage can be quite extensive, particularly for individuals who show signs of persecution feelings.

When sniffed, cocaine constricts the blood vessels of the nose; it can eventually destroy the nose lining. Injected, the drug apparently attacks blood vessels elsewhere in the body and may trigger heart attacks. By no standards—physical, psychological, legal—is cocaine safe.

Amphetamines are the poor man's cocaine. These so-called pep pills produce effects almost identical to those of cocaine. They are sniffed, taken by mouth, or injected. And, yes, they are addicting.

Under a doctor's prescription and management, amphetamines can be useful in reducing weight, fatigue, and depressed-mood complaints. Unfortunately, physicians have handed them out too freely for weight reduction and as antifatigue agents. The pills can reduce weight by cutting down appetite, but they cannot keep you reduced. As time goes by, you need more and more of the drug to keep your appetite under control. Then, too, they do not help you change your long-term eating pattern, which is the most important aspect of any diet program. Pep pills also reduce fatigue but do nothing to help you rearrange your sleep and work habits, which most likely are the actual causative factors of fatigue.

Truckdrivers (half of them, according to one survey) take pep pills to keep awake on long drives. Students use them while cramming for examinations; however, memory is not improved and the pills may give you a false sense of achievement, just as cocaine does. Housewives take them so that they can spring awake in the morning when faced with the chores of house-cleaning. These and countless other casual instances of popping pills are particularly dangerous; "reasons" for taking them seem to proliferate; literally before you know it, you are an addict.

Amphetamine injection—"speed"—can lead to blood-vessel damage. As with any amateur injections there is high risk of infection, hepatitis, allergic reaction, and air bubbles in the blood—any one of which can be lethal. The addiction potential is high, though lower than that of cocaine or heroin. There is no physical dependence, but withdrawal does produce intense craving and fatigue, and depression. Other than withdrawal, there is no known treatment for amphetamine addiction.

Summary: About the only mild stimulant that appears to be "safe" is caffeine in coffee or tea, although some people seem to get hooked on these drinks and have trouble sleeping because of them. Cocaine is a disaster in every way. Pep pills—amphetamines—can be helpful if their consumption is carefully managed by a physician (which is not likely, given the low degree of control that doctors have over their patients) in the treatment of certain mood disorders. Using them illegally on one's own, that is, without prescription, can lead to addiction and to physical damage without commensurate benefits. Of course, not everybody who takes a pep pill is immediately hooked, but if you try it, you may like it; and if you like it, you have thereby increased the risk of addiction. The chances of "liking it" if you take it for "fun" jump up considerably.

As for myself, I drink tea and use behavior-modification methods to fight fatigue. They work.

THE HARD DRUGS. If you are reading this book, the chances are low of your getting involved with opiates, like morphine and heroin, or with methadone. Reason: you are a person who wants to improve himself or herself, and as such your motivation for trying them is low. This is not true of marijuana, barbiturates, and amphetamines, all of which are widespread in our society; you may easily be invited to try one or more of them by a "friend." There are twenty-four million people who have tried marijuana, perhaps an equal number who have used either barbiturates or amphetamines; but only five hundred thousand have taken or are taking any of the opiates. The opiates are used by random groups that are more or less isolated from the mainstream of society. Thus an ordinary person would have to deliberately seek out such a group in order to find not only the opiate, but the social support necessary for trying it. Since he is already part of a larger milieu in which there is ready access to marijuana, barbiturates, and the stimulants, it is not likely that he will take the trouble to find the hard drugs.

Methadone and the opiates produce very little physical damage in either the short or the long run. Indeed, the evidence suggests that these drugs may be safer than alcohol—physically. Small comfort.

Methadone can be obtained legally (by individuals enrolled in programs designed to control heroin addiction); morphine and other opiates, such as codeine, have legal uses as painkillers. Because using heroin—for medical or nonmedical reasons—is always illegal, the user cannot know the dose or purity of the drug, or even if he is getting it at all. Most opiate users favor heroin, injecting it into a vein. This method, especially without knowledge of dose or purity, frequently is the cause of infection, overdose, and allergic reactions, all of which combine to make heroin a more frequent killer than any other drug except alcohol.

The hard drugs are highly addictive, although one, two, or even three attempts will not make an addict, in most instances.

Indeed, the first use will produce nausea and feelings of fear. But, given a socially supportive environment—"friends"—an initiate tries a drug repeatedly; it is not long before he becomes addicted. Then, too, these drugs, unlike cocaine and the amphetamines, produce a physical dependence, which means that if the user attempts to stop, he experiences cramps, diarrhea, headache, and a sense of impending doom. Such withdrawal symptoms serve to reinforce the user's devotion to a way of life that is organized exclusively around drug-taking.

Psychically, hard drugs dull the responses, induce drowsiness, and sharply reduce sex drive. There are cases of long-time morphine users who, under the direction of physicians, are kept on low-level doses and can function with apparently few physical handicaps; however, the reports on these individuals show that they are unable to maintain a lasting interpersonal relationship or stick to any one line of work. In the treatment of heroin addiction, methadone presents a different story: fixed amounts taken orally as a heroin substitute allow the individual to function normally—if his psychic resources were more or less intact before addiction. The fact that methadone itself is addictive makes this methadone-maintenance treatment somewhat less than ideal.

Doctors also use narcotic antagonists to treat heroin addiction. If one of these drugs is taken prior to heroin, all of heroin's "pleasurable" effects are wiped out. Since there is no reinforcement, the habit dies. However, this treatment is effective only if the addict takes the antidrug medicine *every* day; many addicts duck the treatment because taking heroin is so rewarding.

The hard-drug addict has only a slim chance of being cured. Psychological treatment of addiction to heroin, in fact to any drug, must, in my view, be pronounced a failure. There is no evidence that any of the therapeutic communities or rehabilitative programs achieve a higher cure rate than do addicts who are left to their own devices. They certainly do not have as good a record as the methadone programs.

Summary: The hard drugs are powerfully addictive; to keep a habit means a hard life, full of potential danger from the law and from overdose, allergic reaction, poisoning, and infection. In pure form, they are probably safer *physically* than alcohol;

psychically, they can cause devastating changes in personality, sex drive, and general outlook. Treatment for addiction is possible but difficult.

As for myself: not on your life, or even mine!

THE DREAM DRUGS. Substances that produce visions have been known at least since history began. Certain mushrooms, roots, and cactus flowers, if eaten, create distortions of vision, hearing, time, and sense of reality. (Marijuana does these things, but mildly.) Such distortions are hallucinations; hallucinogens are drugs that produce them.

Modern chemistry has added to the store of hallucinogens by extracting the active principles from plant materials, and also by creating entirely new chemicals that are more powerful than anything the plant world has to offer. LSD (lysergic acid diethylamide) is one such new chemical; in an amount equal to a millionth of an ounce, it can change an ordinary person's passing dreams into a phantasmagoria of delight or terror—no one can predict which.

Among the extracted plant materials, the most commonly available (illegally, of course) is mescaline, from cactus; a Mexican species of mushroom yields a drug called psilocybin. They create hallucinations that some users compare to religious exaltation.

Physically, none of the hallucinogens appear to wreak much damage in the short run. At one point it was believed that LSD injured chromosomes and thus might cause defects in the unborn children of LSD users. However, the original research has now been met by counterevidence and the point is in doubt.

Psychically, the hallucinogenic drugs can be substantially damaging (called a "bad trip" by users, a "psychotic episode" by psychiatrists). Some individuals require hospitalization and do not recover for years. Suicides have been reported; so have personality changes—detachment, vagueness—but these have not been widely confirmed. Sometimes the hallucinations appear long after the individual has stopped taking the drug. The risks to a particular individual cannot be predicted, but it is thought that the drugs may be mildly habit-forming: a series of "good" experiences can reinforce the individual's desire to use the drug again. One bad trip may not break the habit; by the time there have been many bad trips the mental damage may be great, even irremediable.

At one time it was claimed that LSD and the other dream drugs induced greater creativity. Careful research has failed to verify this; indeed, art work done under drug influence was judged—by the artist—inferior to that done without the drug. LSD may have some value, as yet unproved, in treating alcohol addiction.

Summary: Hallucinogenic drugs have low physical-damage potential, high psychic-damage risk, modest addiction possibilities. Long-run effects are totally unknown. American Indians and Mexicans have used the drugs for generations. It is impossible to determine at this time how much, if any, of their disease burden —and they have health problems much graver than those of the average white American—is due to the use of hallucinogens.

As for myself: I worry about anything that does something to my brain, which, to me, is my most precious possession. It is the one organ that makes me human. LSD interferes with judgment, which is what we try to educate ourselves to exercise with ever-increasing effectiveness. I guess that in the days when religious visions were important in our society as a source of divine inspiration, the hallucinogenic drugs might have had a place, as they do now in those Indian societies and counterculture groups where visions still play a role. For a modern American attempting to find meaning in an industrial-scientific society, the powers of rationality and judgment are more important than random, un-coordinated hallucinations. Your choice.

OTHER DRUGS. In the never-ending search for drug experience, the people in our drug subculture have turned up an amazing variety of affecting substances, from nutmeg and morning-glory seeds to paint thinner. Even something so apparently harmless as nutmeg can be dangerous. If you use enough of it (a thousand times more than you would put in a pumpkin pie) to effect mental changes, you can end up with serious liver and heart damage. Also on the list are many chemicals that have legitimate medical use, such as tranquilizers, including the two most popularly prescribed, Miltown and Librium.

A doctor uses medicines that carry known bad side effects, including addiction; yet, even equipped with his knowledge, he cannot always avoid undesirable consequences. But at least he is in a good position to do so. The individual who takes drugs on his own has no such safeguard. And, since he is not strict about his dosage, the chances are that bad effects will occur with much higher frequency.

The Last Word

Anybody who takes anything stronger than tea is, in my view, playing against the odds. I realize that for some people, particularly men, playing against odds is a challenge. Racing-car drivers, mountain climbers, football players, for instance, like the sense of danger, the few extra heartbeats that risk generates. They feel, as Ernest Hemingway did in his glorification of the bullfighter, that deliberately to face pain and death is to prove themselves men of superior courage and strength.

There is little one can say to counter such a philosophy except to point out that the benefits—from taking drugs or racing a car—are momentary at best. For me, at least, they would not be sufficient comfort in the likely event of long illness and early death.

9 / How to Drink with Safety, or Something Like Safety

Born to Temperance

"Only bums drink in bars." Thus spoke my father to me, a skinny ten-year-old kid in East Flatbush, Brooklyn, New York, which, circa 1936, could boast only one or two saloons along its main drag, Church Avenue. It was a street of small shops—butchers, bakers, fruit and vegetable stores, hardware, dry goods, and the inevitable candy store with its community telephone ("Run around the corner, kid . . . Shapiro . . . 2B at 401 . . . Telephone for Mrs." And we ran for the two-cent tip). The shortage of saloons (some would say that the market was saturated) was due to the fact that East Flatbush was largely Jewish.

It was only three years after the end of the "great experiment" in which those who marched under the banner of temperance won Prohibition. Lest anyone think that my father walked with them, I must report that he regularly chug-a-lugged a jigger of schnapps before dinner and, for Passover, brought home a gallon of sweet wine, which we never finished. My mother would finally throw it away months later.

In his opinion about bars, my father expressed an attitude toward drinking spirituous liquids that was common among his generation of Jewish immigrants. It was okay for *men* to drink at home in anticipation of food. It was okay to have wine at ceremonial events like Passover, and liquor at weddings and bar mitzvahs—even to get tipsy on such occasions. But to go to a special place like a bar or saloon and drink for the psychic effects of alcohol, or to get drunk by one's self, in short, to make alcohol anything but peripheral in one's life, never.

"Only bums drink in bars." It reverberated through the years . . . so much so that I think I was almost twenty-six before I went into a bar with a friend and had a drink—ginger ale; that despite having chosen the newspaper business, a hard-drinking profession. Drink was a big thing at the late New York *Herald Tribune,* where I passed a quarter of a century of my professional life. One city editor used to say that he didn't trust a reporter who didn't drink. This bit of anonymous doggerel sums it up:

> Sex is the hex of the New York *Times;*
> Drink the ruin of the *Herald Tribune.*

What a clash: Jewish lower-middle-class antidrinking bias smack against the upper-class drinking mores of the *Tribune* stalwarts. Bias won over conformity. After two years in the United States Navy, an institution not noted for its shore-leave sobriety, nothing stronger than Coke ever passed my lips when, as a young reporter, I became part of the normal round of press luncheons, dinners, and cocktail parties.

Enter Alcohol

Nearly six years passed in my marriage before my wife and I served liquor at home. It works as advertised; that is, it makes your guests more voluble, sociable, and easy. Up to that time, we had never known why some of our guests always glanced about like nervous chickens: they were too polite to ask a young married couple for a drink if it didn't appear spontaneously. Even today my drinking is restricted to wine with dinner, perhaps once a week. Occasionally at parties, I will sip a daiquiri (my father never knew what it was). No beer.

Once in my life, I made myself drunk over a disappointment at not receiving a coveted assignment. At home, I would merely have groused; but since I was in San Francisco among hard-drinking, science-writing colleagues, alcohol seemed the manly way out. I am told I am a cheery, whimsical drunk. The next morning fate delivered the assignment along with the most grinding headache I had ever had, a handicap not especially conducive to good work.

Perhaps those who drink regularly will not understand this arm's-length attitude. After all, in America men take hard drinking as a mark of manliness, sexiness, and sophistication. Holding one's liquor is supposed to be a virtue equivalent to batting .400 in the major leagues, and drinking everyone under the table is a feat matched only by knocking out Muhammad Ali. (An interesting aside: prevailing psychiatric opinion holds that an alcoholic drinks to cover latent homosexual drives, that drinking often expresses fears about sexual inadequacy, and that even small amounts of alcohol impair intellectual activity.)

In the same way that drinkers find it hard to understand my feelings about alcohol, I find it hard to accept the central position that drinking occupies in so many people's lives, especially since I know the dangers associated with it. Indeed, I would say that alcohol is the most dangerous drug in America (as I will amply demonstrate). It is also one of the most attractive: as a social instrument it acts as a lubricant; as a psychic instrument it is a tranquilizer. But if abused, its assets quickly become destructive: socially a spoiler, psychically a depressant. Meanwhile, it simultaneously wreaks profound biological damage. I am not anti alcohol; I am anti alcohol abuse—but abuse begins at a far lower level than most Americans are willing to admit.

For the fact is that unless you abstain—as 32 per cent of American adults do—alcohol can easily become, or perhaps is now, a life-threatening substance for you. There is increasing scientific evidence that even so-called social drinking bears risks: alcohol addiction, auto-accident death, liver injury, and the personal, family, and job problems that are generated by abusive drinking. The figures I have show that nine million Americans are in trouble over alcohol. If you do drink, the chances of your getting into trouble with alcohol in your lifetime may be as high as 1 in 6. Of those already committed to hard drinking, 1 in 10 stops, usually for reasons of health, money, job loss, or marriage difficulty.

These figures demonstrate that we are dealing with the most potent substance now currently available on a wide scale.

Most towns have the town drunk; New York, Chicago, and other large American cities have towns of town drunks. They represent the most pathetic end of alcohol addiction. Usually homeless, begging for quarters, subsisting on welfare checks, at the mercy of flophouse marauders, and hopelessly dependent on alcohol, they pass in and out of our courts, jails, and correction camps with the regularity of sunrise and sunset. While indeed these skid-row alcoholics are a serious social problem, in a population of two hundred million Americans they number only one hundred thousand, or less than a tenth of 1 per cent.

The chances of descending to skid row have always been slight for the average drinker, or even heavy drinker. Yet the popular public image of the derelict—as pictured by William Hogarth in his famous set of eighteenth-century drawings—oversimplified the real problem of alcohol among us, even to the point of sweeping the whole nation into the disaster of Prohibition.

Superficially, at least, Prohibition was successful in reducing the number and severity of alcohol disasters. The figures show a sharp reduction in alcohol-related disease between 1919, when the Volstead Act made the manufacture, transport, and sale of alcohol illegal, and 1933, the year of repeal. Many drank bootleg liquor in that "dry" period, perhaps spurred by the thrill of illicit activity, and heavy drinkers continued to drink at the same level, forming the market for the underground alcohol business. Nevertheless, in the fourteen years of illegal liquor, the number of heavy drinkers decreased, along with the rate of alcoholic consumption.

But there is a hypocritical as well as a criminal element that has remained with us as part of the stigma of Prohibition. Those fourteen years also revealed that the specter of dereliction had obscured the fact that problem drinkers existed, throughout all levels of society, in much greater numbers than did derelicts. Some forty years later, this is still true—testifying to the difficulty our society has in facing, let alone dealing with, a problem that requires far more study, patience, and compassion than the mere alarmist extreme reaction of passing a prohibition law. Since 1933 the per-capita consumption of alcohol has climbed dramatically, and with it the number of alcohol-related diseases, including alcoholism.

The Disease Concept

The late Dr. E. M. Jellinek was one of the great authorities on alcoholism, and he, more than any other individual, promoted the concept of alcoholism as a disease. According to Dr. Jellinek's definition of alcoholism—the use of any alcoholic beverage that leads to damage of the individual or society or both—there are about five million alcoholic Americans.

His idea was taken up by Alcoholics Anonymous, a fellowship formed to help the alcoholic achieve sobriety. AA, which claims to have a treatment for all who desire it, defines an alcoholic as "any person whose indulgence in alcohol continuously or periodically results in behavior disruptive of normal relations with his or her work, family or society." To them alcoholism is a disease with a physical susceptibility and a compulsion to drink; and further, they feel that an alcoholic can never allow one sip of alcohol to pass his lips or he will again plummet into darkness. AA believes that once a person becomes an alcoholic, he is so for the rest of his life—sober or not.

The idea of the irretrievability of the alcoholic, the need for him or her to "hit bottom" before he or she can shuck the thralls of alcohol, the mirage of medical treatment, and the disease theory all have—in my view—outlived their usefulness. Aside from introducing some humanity into the handling of the problem drinker, these ideas have not turned around the ever-increasing power of alcohol to enthrall increasing numbers of Americans.

Like the image of the skid-row alcoholic, the concept of alcoholism as a disease may be retarding progress in dealing with the problems of alcohol in our society. Yet the largely successful attempt to describe as sick the individual in trouble over alcohol did for a time improve the situation for individuals with alcohol problems: the concept removed the moralizing over alcohol and brought medical science into the field (with insufficient troops) to replace the battalions of ministers and politicians. Overall, however, the disease concept only modified, but did not eliminate, the inhumane treatment of those with alcohol problems.

The Problem-Drinking Concept

To me alcoholism considered as a disease seems to carry with it a sense of doom so heavy as to exclude the possibility of conquering it through behavior change. I feel that it is healthier, more hopeful, to conceive of alcoholism as "problem drinking."

Dr. Don Cahalan, a research scientist at the University of California at Berkeley, who with his colleagues, Drs. Ira H. Cisin and Helen M. Crossley, has published the most important study on alcohol to date, *The Problem Drinker*, shares my view (rather, I share his):

> It would appear that the concept of alcoholism as a disease has had the undesirable consequences of driving a wedge between the "alcoholic" and society, providing the problem drinker with an alibi for failure to change his behavior and creating an atmosphere in which "alcoholism" becomes a stubborn disease to cure because it is perceived as possessing only the derelict or semi-derelict or the incompetent who is incapable of control over his own behavior.

This could account for the reluctance of many individuals with severe alcohol problems to admit to alcoholism, since to admit you are an alcoholic is to admit you are doomed; only by "hitting bottom" can you ever climb back. "I can always stop when I want" is the defiant cry of the person in trouble over drinking. He cannot face the image of his inexorable descent into dereliction, which the prevailing disease concept engenders.

Yet, as Drs. Cahalan, Cisin, and Crossley discovered in a three-year study, people do change their drinking habits. The study showed that 14 per cent of the people who drink at all are problem drinkers. Of the 87 million American adults who drank in a period of three years, 9.5 million men and 2.6 million women ran into trouble over alcohol. Of these 12 million or so, only half remained problem drinkers for the same period. The rest stopped drinking heavily; they retreated. Alcoholism did not inevitably claim them.

What sorts of problems are we talking about? We are not talking only about the alcoholic as most people picture him or her: lusting after alcohol to the exclusion of all other activity. Rather, we see a person who shows signs of being dependent on alcohol for solving his problems, who drinks to the point where he often suffers from physical aftermath, who is frequently drunk, who may be in trouble with drinking on the job or at home, or whose health is impaired.

If you are a man who drinks at all, the chances of your ending up with a significant drinking problem are 1 in 4; if you are a drinking woman, the chances are 1 in 10. Those are mighty high odds. The reason we do not perceive as much problem drinking around as these odds would lead us to expect is that the problems occur to different people at different times. Then, too, many individuals have the financial means to hide the fact that they are in trouble with drink. And finally, many problems—repeated drunkenness, for example—may not be seen as problems.

Alcohol and Physical Health

Can alcohol lower your chances of living out your biologically given life span? Few would doubt that the answer is yes. Alcohol snips off years in two ways: it acts directly to poison your organs, and it increases your risk of accidents, particularly automobile, by impairing your reactions and judgments.

Dr. Raymond Pearl, of Johns Hopkins University, discovered the shortened life span of drinkers in 1926. A thirty-year-old man who drinks moderately or not at all will live eight years longer than a heavy drinker of the same age. Eight years is a long, long time. Today the nondrinker of thirty can expect to live to seventy-six, a heavy drinker to sixty-eight, or, put another way, he will enjoy his retirement for only three years. Yet he may not enjoy it at all, because the toll on his health from alcohol could make the last years miserable.

Dr. Charles Lieber, of Mount Sinai Hospital in New York, has shown that what many drinkers would consider moderate consumption of alcohol—two drinks a day—causes fatty deposits in the livers of healthy and well-fed bodies. That alcohol is toxic to the liver, irrespective of the drinker's health, was an important discovery. Previously, most scientists supposed that poor eating habits brought on by the alcoholic's way of life produced the biological damage. Prior to World War II, many skid-row dere-licts turned up at hospitals with pellagra, a vitamin-deficiency disease. Since the war, bread has been vitamin-enriched and pellagra among the skid-row denizens has all but disappeared. But pneumonia, brain damage, heart disease, hardening of the liver, and bleeding throat veins still persist among these men and other heavy drinkers.

It used to be that physicians would prescribe a cocktail or a glass of wine or beer for men who had had a heart attack, reason-ing that the drink was tranquilizing and also increased blood flow in the coronary arteries. A series of tests showed that alcohol—in amounts equal to a single cocktail, glass of wine, or can of beer—decreases the efficiency of a damaged heart. There is a strong movement in medical circles to eliminate this ancient prescription for heart victims.

Heavy drinking has been connected to heart-muscle damage, but the evidence is not so strong for that as it is for damage to the liver. It is the hardening of the liver that causes, among other symptoms, hemorrhaging in the throat. There is also suggestive evidence that alcohol in combination with cigarette-smoking may trigger cancer of the throat, but the connection is far from proved.

Alcohol and Accidents

Alcohol efficiently sends you to your Maker by causing acci-dents. There is no question that a drink before starting on an automobile ride can be your passage to the cemetery when you least expect it. No matter what you have come to believe about your ability to "hold your liquor," alcohol impairs your ability to drive a car. Driving is a complex co-ordination of muscular reaction, observation, and learned behavior. Recent studies indi-cate that even one drink can impair human capacity in those areas.

Of the fifty thousand auto deaths a year in this country, it is believed that alcohol contributes to more than half. One re-searcher found that half the drivers killed in crashes had more alcohol in their blood than the average man arrested for drunken-ness. Another discovered that a disturbing number of people arrested for drunken driving could be defined psychiatrically as alcoholics and no amount of punishment—jail, revocation of license, or fine—could stop them from drinking and then driving. Most scary is a statistic revealing that the worst drunk-accident records were found among those who drink only once a month— social drinkers.

When you consider that alcohol is implicated in at least half of the fifty thousand highway deaths and half of the 1.8 million disabling injuries and the $8.9 billion in property damage, wages lost, and medical expenses brought on by highway accidents each year, it becomes clear that we are not talking about a fun beverage. The alcohol industry likes to refer to drunken driving as a "people problem, not a product problem," implying that if only people used alcohol more sanely, we would not have that awful toll. Nonsense. It is in the nature of alcohol, given our social attitudes toward drinking—fostered by the alcohol industry itself—that it will trap a significant number of people into addictive drinking, problem drinking, and heavy drinking. Those trapped will drive automobiles and kill and be killed.

Teetotalers All?

It is not the aim of this book to deal with the problem of changing the drinking habits of a Dionysian society into those of the meditative, moderative, work-oriented Apollonian. Nor have I listed the risks of a drinking career in order to make us a nation of teetotalers. But what we do have to recognize is that there are many individuals among us who run a high risk of turning alcohol into a problem. We are just beginning to identify them and the conditions that raise the risks above the tolerable level.

Why People Drink

In order to arrive at a practical theory of why people drink alcohol, it is first necessary to limn the contributions of three key forces, as noted by Dr. Jellinek: biology, psychology, society. It might then be possible to see what has to be changed in each of the three conditions in order to modify human behavior.

It is clear that the potential combinations of hereditary factors create a unique biochemistry for each individual on this planet. Those combinations express themselves in the multitudinous human sizes, shapes, colors, and intelligences. While human beings generally have the same recognizable outline, it is remarkable that the incidence of look-alikes (twins excepted) is so low. The well-known diversity of fingerprints points to underlying chemical differences, in degree if not in kind.

Physicians have long known that individuals respond idiosyncratically to drugs. Give one person a tranquilizer and his mental fog clears as if the hot sun of reason shone on it; give the same chemical to another, and he breaks out in a rash that makes him as unhappy as his mental state. Thus we should not be surprised to find out that individuals respond to alcohol in biologically different ways. It is known that if you give three ounces of 100-proof whisky to seven persons, you can easily get seven different behavioral reactions: one will get sleepy, another aggressive, a third talkative, a fourth weepy, and so on. But in the way the body responds to alcohol, few *chemical* differences among individuals have been found.

Alcoholics Anonymous literature speaks of alcoholics as "allergic" to alcohol. But nobody has been able to identify such a reaction according to AA's definition, that is, a special sensitivity to the addictive properties of alcohol on a biological basis. Some individuals will show a blotchy, pink skin after a drink or two, but that reaction seems in no way related to the AA addiction sensitivity.

Dr. Roger Williams, of the University of Texas, carried out numerous experiments in animals to show that a vitamin deficiency could lead animals to drink more alcohol. He hoped to find a similar vitamin deficiency in human beings susceptible to alcohol addiction, to discover a biochemical profile that would be as unique to each individual as his fingerprint, and finally to uncover the alcoholic biochemical profile. Alas, no such vitamin deficiency or alcoholic profile has been established.

Similarly, thirty years ago scientists reported hormone deficiencies that were linked with a craving for alcohol. Recently, however, Dr. Jack Mendelsohn and his associates at Harvard Medical School pinned most of the nutritional and hormonal deficiencies of heavy drinkers to the effects of alcohol on the organs after a lifetime of drinking. The deficiencies did not produce craving for drink.

A recent report suggests that the human body creates from alcohol a substance similar to morphine. If confirmed, the finding is of great theoretical importance; however, it shifts the question of alcohol addiction to understanding the biological ground for morphine addiction, another biochemical mystery.

If there is a biological-chemical underpinning to alcohol addiction or habit, it eludes the most sensitive tools of science. One thing is clear: for most individuals alcohol produces pleasant mental effects. Those pleasant effects are certainly dependent upon the response of nerves to the drug, even though the mechanics of the response on a chemical level are unknown. In this sense there does exist a biological underpinning: alcohol is rewarding and as such is a powerful habit former.

If it could be established that, because of biological differences, certain individuals are more sensitive to the rewarding properties of alcohol, it might be possible to identify such persons in advance and warn them off alcohol, as we now warn diabetics off sugar. But that is a hope for the future.

For some time psychologists and psychiatrists have been attempting to reconstruct the psychological history of the problem drinker in order to find some psychological basis for his current drinking. Yet, as in the case of drug-addiction studies, there is no way of determining which psychological features come from drinking and which were there before heavy drinking began. Thus it was possible for the psychologists and psychiatrists to weave their own theories, depending on what part of the personality each attributed to current drinking and what to pre-existing psychology.

Let us look at just one of these reports. Dr. Israel Zwerling, of the Albert Einstein College of Medicine in New York, examined forty-six male problem drinkers and extracted a constellation of specific psychological traits. In short, this was the alcoholic personality:

1. Schizoid, that is, showing a "basic sense of estrangement or separateness from people, of withdrawal from close interpersonal relationships";

2. Dependent in that they "achieve security through the efforts of others";

3. Depressed, with a basic sense of futility, self-loathing, and sadness;

4. Hostile, with marked evidence of chronic rage, although overt behavior is not violent;

5. Sexually immature. Often they are unable to establish a masculine identification. Their heterosexual activity is much reduced, with symptoms of impotency and even active homosexuality.

Dr. Zwerling was, however, observing the full-blown alcoholic —the average man in his study had had problems with drinking for at least nineteen years. I can look at each of the characteristics suggested by Dr. Zwerling and see them as formed by the mill of years of hard drinking and alcohol dependency. Who would not, after nineteen years of trouble that brings you into conflict with society, family, and friends, be depressed with a "basic sense of futility, self-loathing, and sadness"?

One thorough review of the psychiatric literature concluded that there was no defined alcoholic personality. Certainly, a psychiatric study is inadequate in determining what personality traits lead to alcohol addiction or problems. Additional information is necessary about a large number of drinkers and non-drinkers—data concerning economic class, ethnic background, education, personal habits, attitudes, drinking patterns—gathered at different times of their lives over a period of several years. Only then would it be possible to determine which factors are predisposing.

The CCC study (conducted by Drs. Cahalan, Cisin, and Crossley) has done just that. In 1964 and 1965 the researchers sent out interviewers to talk to 2,450 Americans chosen at random. In 1967, they reinterviewed 1,400 of them. And in 1973, 1,400 were to be interviewed again. Important data about the kinds of people who drink heavily and who get into trouble over alcohol has already come from this study, which also provides important information about the social conditions that produce drinking problems.

With the information from the CCC study we are in a position to assess your risk of getting into trouble over alcohol. Instead of summarizing that material now, which I think would spoil the effectiveness of the assessment for you, I am going to ask you to first fill out a number of short questionnaires that follow. The answers will determine your risk of getting into trouble over alcohol. Then we will discuss their meaning.

I should add here a note of caution: because the studies of alcohol in society are in their infancy, the data are at best suggestive rather than definitive. As you go through the rest of the chapter, determining your risk of getting into trouble over alcohol, keep in mind that a "high risk" score is merely a warning sign, not a sentence of doom. The numerical estimates were derived from studies of populations and when I apply them to individuals, I am taking a leap that is not entirely justified. But since these materials are really the only instruments we have, they are at the moment better than none. Inasmuch as Drs. Cahalan, Cisin, and Crossley did not intend to use their data for individual assessment of risk, I must take the responsibility for presenting the material in this form. I have simplified it considerably and made certain assumptions in scoring that are not fully proved. Nevertheless, I believe the risk scores are useful.

Determining Your Risk

As with all behavior that has to do with health, the rational approach is to determine what benefit you get from a particular behavior and what risk that behavior produces for threatening your life. For example, despite the fact that 50,000 people die on the highways each year, and 1.8 million suffer disabling injuries, we all continue to drive. We have reckoned that the benefits we get from the automobile far outweigh the chance of suffering accident or death. Of course, many people simply do not rationally carry out the calculation. In some way they have convinced themselves that they are invulnerable to automobile injury. Similarly, there are those heavy drinkers who have decided that they are invulnerable to its addictive and health-impairing powers.

One of the ingredients in determining risk is, of course, how much you drink. A current myth in American life holds that "good" liquor cannot hurt you. Another myth is the one about the eighty-year-old man who drank a fifth of bourbon every day of his life and it never hurt him. There is also the ubiquitous three-martini lunch that "I'm used to." None of these can be taken seriously in the face of the growing scientific evidence that how much you drink affects your life.

What counts in drinking is the amount of alcohol actually taken in, not necessarily what it's mixed with. An ounce of hard liquor—about 90 proof—has the same amount of alcohol in it as a four-ounce glass of wine, which has the same alcohol content as a twelve-ounce glass of beer. (People do get drunk on beer.) So it almost doesn't matter what you drink; servings of liquor, wine, and beer equal each other.

In the table below circle the number next to the statement that most closely indicates how often you drink at least one serving of any alcohol-containing beverage: beer, wine, bourbon, rum, Scotch, brandy, cordial, or whatever. A serving is one ounce of hard liquor or its equivalent.

Drinking Frequency

1. Three times a day
2. Twice a day
3. Once a day
4. Nearly every day
5. Three to four times a week
6. Once or twice a week
7. Two to three times a month
8. Once a month
9. Less than once a month
10. Less than once a year or never

You have established how *often* you drink. Now you have to determine how *much* you drink each time. To do that, answer the next questions by circling the letter that best describes what you do:

QUESTION ONE: Many people have *five* or *six* drinks at a sitting. How frequently do you have five or six drinks?

A. Nearly every time
B. More than half the time
C. Less than half the time

D. Once in a while
E. Never

QUESTION TWO: Many people drink *three* or *four* drinks on each occasion; how about you? Circle the letter that best describes what you do.

F. Nearly every time
G. More than half the time
H. Less than half the time
I. Once in a while
J. Never

QUESTION THREE: Many people drink *one* or *two* drinks on each occasion. When you drink, how often do you take one or two drinks?

K. Nearly every time
L. More than half the time
M. Less than half the time
N. Once in a while
O. Never

Heavy Drinker, Moderate Drinker, Light Drinker?

Using the answers so far, you can now determine if you are a heavy, moderate, or light drinker. The definitions come from the CCC study. (My wife would say that anybody who drank once a day would be a heavy drinker.) The CCC study created the divisions, partly because they saw that their definition of heavy drinkers carried the greatest social risk. To determine what kind of drinker you are, follow the instructions for Scoring Your Drinking.

Scoring Your Drinking

Recall that on the appropriate table you circled a number to indicate how often you drink alcohol. You will find the same numbers and headings below. Look for the one you selected. Under each heading you will find three categories: light, moderate, and heavy drinker and under those labels you will see letters. Some letters appear alone, others in combination. Those letters represent your answers to the three questions about the *amount* of alcohol you drink.

Note that E, J, and O do not appear. They do not count. AX means A alone or in combination with any other letter; similarly for BX, CX, et cetera.

Now look for the combination of letters represented by your answers to find the type of drinker you are.

No. 1: *Three Times a Day*

> If you take as little as one drink every time you drink during the day, you are classified as a heavy drinker. There are no moderate or light drinkers who drink three times a day.

No. 2: *Twice a Day*

Heavy Drinker	Moderate Drinker	Light Drinker
AX, BX, CX, DX, FX, GX, KH, LH	KI, LI, K, L	None

No. 3: *Once a Day*

Heavy Drinker	Moderate Drinker	Light Drinker
AX, BX, CX, DX, FX, GX	KH, LH, KI, LI	K, L

No. 4: *Nearly Every Day*

Heavy Drinker	Moderate Drinker	Light Drinker
AX, BX, CX, DX, FX, GX	KH, LH, KI, LI	K, L

No. 5: *Three to Four Times a Week*

Heavy Drinker	Moderate Drinker	Light Drinker
AX, BX, C, CF, CG, CH, CI, CM, CN, F, FM, FN, G, GM, GN	CK, CL, D, DK, DL, KH, KL	KI, K, L, LI

No. 6: *Once or Twice a Week*

Heavy Drinker	Moderate Drinker	Light Drinker
AX, BX, C, CF, CG, CH, CI, CM, CN	F, FM, FN, G, GM, GN, CK, CL, D, DK, DL, KH, KL	KI, K, L, LI

No. 7: *Two to Three Times a Month*

Heavy Drinker	Moderate Drinker	Light Drinker
AX, BX	C, CF, CG, CH, CI, CM, CN, CK, CL, D, DK, DL, DG, DH, F, FM, FN, G, GM, GN	K, KH, KI, L, LH, LI

No. 8: *Once a Month*

Heavy Drinker	Moderate Drinker	Light Drinker
None	AX, BX, CX, DF, DG, F, FM, FN, G, GM, GN	D, DK, DL, K, KH, KI, L, LH, LI

No. 9: *Less than Once a Month*

If you drink less than once a month, you are classified as an infrequent drinker.

No. 10: *Less than Once a Year or Never*

Anybody in this category is called an abstainer.

If your combination of letters cannot be found in the table, there is something inconsistent about how you answered the questions. For example: IM would mean that you drink three or four drinks *once in a while* and you drink one or two drinks *less than half the time*. That leaves something less than half the time unaccounted for.

IF YOU ARE A HEAVY DRINKER. If you're a heavy drinker, the chances are something like 8 out of 10 that you will get into trouble over alcohol.

Typical heavy drinkers are those who drink at least one drink three times a day, *or*

drink three or four drinks more than half the time and who drink at least once a day, *or*

drink six or seven drinks more than half the time and who drink at least twice a month, *or*

range between three and six drinks on the average and drink once or twice a week.

Perhaps this doesn't seem like much to you; after all, many of your friends drink about what you do and do not seem to be in trouble . . . now. But the CCC investigation clearly pinpoints that such heavy drinking means trouble. More than that, the amounts of alcohol involved are more than sufficient to cause the biological changes in the liver and heart that have been detected in various careful studies.

If you circled A or B, that is, if you drink five or six drinks at a time, even if you do it once a month and are classified as a moderate drinker, your risk of future trouble is quite high. If you drink that much at one sitting, you probably will get drunk, and drunkenness is counted as being in trouble over alcohol. Of all the groups studied by CCC, this sort of binge drinking—five or six drinks at a time—seemed to be the most dangerous and predictive of difficulties ahead.

If you drink three or more times a day, even though you may take as little as one drink each time, you may be well along in the habit-forming stage. Three beers, three glasses of wine, or three cocktails does not sound like much until you consider that each drink means four to eight sips. Each sip is a reward. So if you drink three times a day every day, you are being rewarded at least 4,400 times a year with a very powerful drug.

Two drinks a day would not be too bad if you could keep it at that level. However, as with all mood-changing drugs, the body will in time require more alcohol to get the same mood change and you may find that the amount you take each day will slowly increase. If you are taking two a day now, you probably were taking one a day not too many years ago; in a few years you may find that you are up to three or more a day, with some days certainly at four.

The typical situation begins with the martini before dinner at home. Then you find that two martinis seem even better. Then on some days, you have a drink for lunch. And in a few years, it is two drinks for lunch, two for dinner, and a nightcap—and you are up to the level of the very heaviest drinkers. And the chances are the drug-taking is a habit. How strong a habit depends on other factors, which we will explore.

Incidentally, the scenario could be repeated with beer or wine; it is the amount of alcohol and the frequency that count, not what it is mixed with.

IF YOU ARE A MODERATE DRINKER. A typical moderate drinker is one who drinks twice a day and has at least one drink, *or* drinks nearly every day and has one or two drinks every time and sometimes as many as four, *or*

drinks once or twice a week and has three or four drinks every time, *or*

drinks twice or three times a month with three or four drinks every time and sometimes as many as five or six.

If you fall into this category, you will notice that you are not terribly far behind the heavy drinker; indeed, there is a suggestion that the moderate drinker has a high risk of going on to become a heavy drinker. That does not mean that the progression is inexorable, merely that the risk is high. The same arguments apply: regular drinking or drinking large amounts, even if infrequently, can be habit-forming; tolerance can take over and you may escalate to get the same effects; the amount of alcohol taken by a moderate drinker is sufficient to produce liver and heart damage.

Sure, if you could maintain your drinking pattern at two drinks a day, you would have little to worry about. At that level both the biological damage and the susceptibility to habituation may be quite small. But again, the rewarding mechanism and the tendency of the body to build tolerance may throw your drinking into the heavy category. Each year about 10 per cent of moderate drinkers become heavy drinkers. Fortunately, an almost equal number of heavy drinkers cut back, too.

IF YOU ARE A LIGHT DRINKER. The typical light drinker is a person who drinks once a day but has one or two drinks, never more, *or*

drinks three or four times a week and has one or two drinks and sometimes as many as three or four, *or*

drinks one to two times a month and takes one or two drinks but will have as many as five or six on occasion.

The light drinker only occasionally gets into trouble over alcohol. His intake is such that the risk of biological damage is low, unless he is already ill with another disease—such as coronary heart disease—when even the small amount of alcohol represented in light drinking may be damaging.

The important thing to watch, of course, is whether the amount and frequency are increasing. Do you find yourself drinking three drinks a day when just a few months ago you never had more than two? That is escalation and it may mean that you are graduating into the moderate-drinking class. Again: such increases are not inexorable; only the risk is there, proportionately lower for the light drinker than for the moderate and heavy drinkers.

American Drinkers

The CCC studies discovered how Americans shape up as drinkers. The breakdown is as follows:

Heavy	12 per cent
Moderate	13 per cent
Light	28 per cent
Infrequent	15 per cent
Abstainers	32 per cent

You can see at once that drinking is a very common activity. The majority of Americans (53 per cent) drink regularly, two out of three Americans can be classified as drinkers—which means that teetotalers are in the minority.

Incidentally, with all the brouhaha over the other drugs in this country, it is interesting to note that 85 per cent of all Americans have had an alcoholic drink before the age of eighteen. No other mood-changing drug has been so widely used by adolescents. In addition, more than a third of the youngsters under sixteen drink alcohol in some form regularly and more than half of these young people have had alcohol away from home. In other words, half of American youth have had alcohol *illegally;* this is a greater proportion than those who have had marijuana.

I only point this out to show that with such a common, approved, commercialized, and, in certain ways, beneficial drug it would be impossible to wipe it out. But it is curious that the American public will stand for the risks of alcohol. After all, cyclamates—the artificial sweeteners—were banned because they gave a few rats cancer at dose levels fifty times that taken by human beings. Alcohol kills human beings and we do little about it. But you can.

An Alcohol Risk Test

Now I am going to ask you to take a test that will give you some idea of the risk you run of getting into trouble over alcohol. I will tell you later what that trouble is likely to be. A few of the questions below have shown some power to pick out people who will run into difficulty. Others do not. Do not try to guess which ones they are; simply answer the questions truthfully if you want an estimate about yourself.

Just circle agree or disagree after each statement below according to whether it represents a true statement about you or your opinions. Do not skip any questions. Answer them as best you can.

A. I am often bothered by nervousness.	Agree	Disagree
B. My father* never had more than two or three drinks at a time.	Agree	Disagree
C. My father* used to have four and sometimes more drinks occasionally.	Agree	Disagree
D. When I drink I feel sleepy.	Agree	Disagree
E. Compared with two years ago, conditions in my life have grown worse.	Agree	Disagree
F. It is okay for me to take eight drinks if I want to.	Agree	Disagree
G. It is okay for me to take four drinks if I want to.	Agree	Disagree
H. I drink because I like the taste.	Agree	Disagree
I. My close friends do not come from my neighborhood.	Agree	Disagree
J. If I had to give up drinking, I would miss it a lot.	Agree	Disagree
K. I always finish things I start, even if they are not very important.	Agree	Disagree
L. If I had my choice, I would live my life very differently.	Agree	Disagree
M. Good things can be said about drinking.	Agree	Disagree

N. I am somewhat overweight.	Agree	Disagree
O. I was raised in a town with more than 5,000 population.	Agree	Disagree
P. I am very satisfied with having reached my life's goals.	Agree	Disagree
Q. I have the feeling I am different.	Agree	Disagree
R. My father* disapproved of drinking.	Agree	Disagree
S. Sometimes I feel so lonesome.	Agree	Disagree
T. Nearly every time I am with close friends we have drinks.	Agree	Disagree
U. I drink to celebrate special occasions.	Agree	Disagree
V. It is important for me to drink to be sociable.	Agree	Disagree
W. I find it hard to deal with people because I don't know what to expect.	Agree	Disagree
X. Very few of my close friends drink a lot.	Agree	Disagree
Y. I don't belong to any organizations.	Agree	Disagree

* If your father died when you were very young answer this question about the man who was head of your household when you were growing up. If there was no such man, answer it about your mother.

Scoring Your Risk

Again keep in mind that the scores are purely suggestive; I extracted these scores—rather crudely—from studies of populations by Dr. Cahalan and his colleagues. Those studies themselves did not account for the whole story on the risk of drinking. A high-risk score is not an occasion for panic, but should give you pause for a sober (!) assessment of your current drinking pattern.

Obviously if you do not drink at all, your risk is nil; if you drink moderately or heavily, as I have described, then your risk is higher. However, not all moderate or heavy drinkers get into trouble. The test above tells you whether you as a moderate or heavy drinker (and in some cases as a light drinker) are headed for difficulty over drinking. Here, you are going to score yourself by groups of questions; each group represents a different kind of risk.

Group One:

F. Agree, score 1 point
G. Agree, score 1 point
J. Agree, score 1 point
M. Agree, score 1 point
V. Agree, score 1 point

If you scored 3 or more, you have a high risk; 1 to 2, medium risk; 0, low risk. The group-one questions relate to your attitudes toward drinking. A high score means that you approve of drinking and in particular you approve of heavy drinking. Studies show that people who approve of drinking and who themselves drink heavily or moderately have a high risk of getting into trouble over alcohol.

Group Two:

C. Agree, score 1 point
R. Disagree, score 1 point
T. Agree, score 1 point
X. Disagree, score 1 point

If you scored a 3 or 4, your risk is high; 1 to 2, medium risk; 0, low risk. This group measures the degree to which drinking is approved in your social circle now and as you were growing up. Again, being brought up among people who drink heavily and who approve of drinking raises the possibility of your drinking heavily and also of getting into trouble over alcohol. Certain ethnic groups—Irish, English, Latins, black males—all grow up under such conditions, and study after study finds that these groups have the most trouble with alcohol. People brought up in the Bible Belt of America or according to Jewish, Chinese, or Italian mores do not frequently have such difficulties, because either all drinking is disapproved of or only light drinking is allowed.

Group Three:

A. Agree, score 1 point
L. Agree, score 1 point
S. Agree, score 1 point
W. Agree, score 1 point

The score: 3 or 4 is high risk; 1 or 2, medium risk; 0, low risk. The group-three score tells you how psychologically disturbed you may be. If you agree with all the statements, you are a person beset by nervousness, loneliness, fears of social difficulty, and a desire to start all over again. A high score here is not so powerfully predictive of trouble over alcohol as are high scores in groups one and two. This finding conforms with the difficulty psychiatrists have had in discovering the alcohol-prone personality. Essentially, then, it is the social controls or lack of them, rather than psychological problems as almost everybody has believed, that lead into difficulty over alcohol.

Group Four:
I. Agree, score 1 point
O. Agree, score 1 point
Y. Agree, score 1 point
If you're single, separated, or divorced, score 1 point.

The score: 3 to 4, high risk; 1 to 2, medium risk; 0, low risk. This group estimates the amount of social control exerted on you. A high score indicates that you have fewer ties to others than most Americans; thus you will tend to drink more and be more susceptible to getting into difficulty. Group four is as powerful a predictor of alcohol risk as groups one and two.

Group Five:
E. Agree, score 1 point
P. Disagree, score 2 points

The score: 3, high risk; 1 to 2, medium risk; 0, low risk. If you have a high score here, you have unfavorable expectations in your life. You are dissatisfied and you see things getting worse. Under such conditions, heavy drinking will contribute to a high possibility of getting into trouble over alcohol. Incidentally, all the other questions are dummies; they have little or no predictive value.

YOUR OVERALL RISK. Of course, if you score high in each group of questions, watch out: you may be heading for trouble. If, in addition, you drink for dramatic mood change, then you bear an additional burden of risk. Naturally, most people drink because they like the mood-changing effects of alcohol; there are also many who like the taste or who do it to be sociable. The person who scores high in the questionnaire and who drinks for psychological escape may be most at risk. Typically, such a person will drink many drinks at one sitting even though he or she may fall into the moderate-drinking class. To repeat: these tests were derived from questionnaires answered by the population at large. Statistically, the scores are not strong predictors for individuals, only for groups; therefore, in looking at your risk scores think of them as indicators of risk rather than as absolute predictions.

The Kinds of Trouble

When you think of somebody in trouble over alcohol you may visualize the town drunk, the skid-row alcoholic, or the guy who comes to work every morning with a hangover. You may also be familiar with the list of questions given out by Alcoholics Anonymous to test people on their difficulty with alcohol. If so, you may see the alcoholic as a person who has lost control and whose craving for alcohol inexorably leads him to doom. But, as I have noted earlier, for the majority of people in America that is not true. Among the heavy drinkers, about 1 in 10 is truly addicted to the drug in the sense that most of the medical profession and AA see it. For that group, who may number a million Americans, this book has nothing to offer. Let us discuss the majority of people headed for trouble over alcohol.

You are in trouble over alcohol if you find yourself psychologically dependent on drinking and have four or more drinks at a sitting. You are psychologically dependent if you answer yes to three or more of the following questions:

1. Do you find it *very helpful* to have a drink—a highball, cocktail, some wine or beer—when you are depressed and nervous?

2. Is it *very important* for you to drink when you want to forget your worries?

3. Is it *very important* for you to have a drink to cheer you up when you are in a bad mood?

4. Is it *very important* for you to drink when you are tense?

Actually there are degrees of psychological dependence. If you answer yes to all the questions you are most dependent, as are less than 1 per cent of adults in America. If you answer yes to one *or more* of these questions, then you have 15 per cent of American adults to keep you company. Being psychologically dependent on drink is to be in one kind of trouble, and it is an important kind of trouble because, more than any other, it predicts that alcohol will cause you problems in other areas of your life.

A second kind of trouble is symptomatic drinking. To find out if you exhibit symptomatic-drinking behavior, answer the following questions yes or no:

1. Have you recently taken a drink to get rid of a hangover?

2. Recently, if you started drinking has it been difficult for you to stop before becoming completely intoxicated?

3. Did you wake up the next day unable to remember the things you did while drinking?

4. Have you been skipping a number of regular meals because of drinking?

5. Are you tossing down several drinks pretty fast to get a quicker effect from them?

6. Do you take a quick drink or so when no one is looking?

7. Do you take a few quick drinks before going to a party to make sure you have enough?

Anybody who answers yes to one or more of these items has been drinking at least four drinks at a sitting recently. Thirteen per cent of American adults could answer yes to one or more of the above questions.

If you add the score for psychological dependency to the score for symptomatic drinking you get an even better prediction of your chances of being in trouble in other areas.

Other Troubles

Are you intoxicated frequently? That is: Do you take five or more drinks on four or more days a week . . . or take eight or twelve drinks somewhat less frequently? Or do you get high or tight between one and three times a month? Or do you do something in between, that is, take five or more drinks once, twice, or three times a week? Then you have trouble with intoxication. Twelve per cent of Americans have that trouble.

Are your relatives and friends giving you a hard time over your drinking? For example, has your wife or husband said you ought to cut down? That if you did not stop you would not have a marriage? Have your neighbors warned you about your drinking? Eleven per cent of Americans have had trouble with relatives over their drinking and 6 per cent have been warned by neighbors and friends. Of course, some have had both.

Something like five million people, 4.5 per cent of the 110 million adults have had trouble on the job. Perhaps half a million people lost or nearly lost their jobs. Of the rest, some were told to cut down, went to work drunk, or got high during working hours.

One person in ten reports health problems over drinking. Almost half of them have been told by doctors to cut down on drinking. That means five million people have been asked by their physicians to reduce the amount that they drink. That is trouble.

And, while we think of alcohol as a social lubricant, there are many in our society for whom alcohol causes belligerence. One person in ten reports that alcohol makes him aggressive, and something like three hundred thousand people a year actually get into a fight over drink. Incidentally, that tendency to fight after drinking could account for almost half the murders in this country.

Finally, a lot of people—6.5 per cent—find that drinking harms their pocketbook, either because they spend too much money on drinking or because it takes them away from earning money.

Overall, we are talking about many people in trouble. If we combine the various troubles into a problem score, as Drs. Cahalan, Cisin, and Crossley have done, then it turns out that 9 per cent of American adults have what might be called severe problems with alcohol. That 9 per cent represents about ten to twelve million adults. And the question is, are you among them now or heading for membership in that group?

It should be obvious to you that your risk of trouble over alcohol depends to a great extent on the response of the people around you to your drinking pattern. If your family or friends think nothing of your getting drunk on weekends, then the chances are that your risk score will be low. On the other hand, if I got drunk on weekends, my wife would be pushing me to go see a doctor. This interaction between you and society is what makes assessment of risk from alcohol so difficult and is why your risk scores should be taken only as indicators.

By now you should have a picture of yourself in relation to alcohol. You know your pattern of drinking—that is, how much and how often—your risk of getting into trouble based on your answers to the risk tests, and whether you are in trouble over alcohol now, and, if not, the kinds of troubles you face if your risk is high. As I have said frequently, a high risk does not mean that you will become an alcoholic. Even if you exhibit psychological dependence or symptomatic drinking, both highly related to other troubles, that does not mean you are headed for skid row. There are literally millions of people who do go along for years with symptomatic drinking, and even psychological dependence, and get no better and no worse. I would not want to live that way myself, and such difficulties take their financial, personal, and health tolls, but those millions do not "hit bottom." Many stop drinking as they get older; others die early from drinking-related causes, such as accident or liver damage.

There is one comment to be made at this point. It used to be believed that alcohol was largely an old man's problem. Again, we always looked at the end result of many years of drinking, at those people who came to the attention of the police or hospitals. Such persons were likely to be older and poorer than the rest of us because they no longer had the financial and physical resources to maintain high levels of drinking or to cover up the troubles that drink got them into.

However, if you look at free-living men and women, as the CCC study did, then you will find that it is young men between twenty-one and twenty-four who have the most trouble with alcohol—as we have defined trouble, that is, symptomatic drinking, psychological dependence, intoxication, warnings from family and friends. Indeed, it is Dr. Cahalan's guess that there is even more trouble in the age group from seventeen to twenty-one. In that case, alcohol is a young person's problem just as much as an older person's, perhaps more.

To Reduce Risk

Now, how do you reduce risk from drinking? Immediately it must occur to you that one simply drinks less. How much less? For most people it means setting a limit of two drinks a day, preferably less. Why two? It is at this level that one begins to see liver damage, the highest degree of binge drinking, and intoxication. This is contrary to the advice generally given about drinking up to now. Most alcohol experts and those in AA have said that people with alcohol problems are alcoholics and should not drink at all. Again, that advice has been based on observations of people strongly addicted to alcohol who cannot—in the main—return to social drinking. The statistics indicate, however, that many heavy drinkers do cut back on their own.

The two-drink-a-day limit is a limit, not a goal. If you are drinking less than that now, you do not have to prove your manliness or your female sophistication by increasing your drinking to that level. If you drink more than two drinks a day, you may be heading for trouble.

If you drink to ease your troubles, don't. Here we have the same problem as with food. Many people eat to calm themselves. The thing to do is attack the problem by giving yourself another way of dealing with personal difficulty. But you have to do it at the moment when the trouble stimulus appears. For example: suppose you have a fight with your boss just before lunchtime. You can hardly wait to get to the corner bar to get that drink. Here is where you use behavior modification. First, turn off all thoughts of drink. If you cannot, you must conjure up some dreadful image that will do it: a picture of the skid-row bum, an incapacity to have sex, bleeding in your throat. Then have some alternative behavior ready: talking to a colleague at work, buckling down to what you normally do, telephoning your spouse or a friend. In other words, at the moment when you would normally turn to drink, turn to people. You can use the same technique to limit your drinking when you are in a social situation. The turning off of the stimulus that leads you to order that second or third drink can be accomplished by the use of mental images. Furthermore, if you drink very, very slowly, you will drink less and less for the mood-changing power of alcohol and more for its socially lubricating effect. Fast drinking simply means that you get a high concentration of alcohol in your blood and brain, and that can lead to tolerance and addiction.

Do not binge. Getting drunk and staying drunk for a day or two appears to be among the most dangerous activities of drinking. It not only leads to automobile accidents, it also seems to be one of the best predictors of further troubles with alcohol. Binge drinking seems to be related to the type of friends you have. If you go out with "the boys" to have a good time by getting drunk and staying drunk, you will find it harder and harder to refuse their invitations. The best suggestion I have is: change your friends or find some way of turning down binge parties.

Try to see alcohol as a dangerous drug whose use in small amounts may be harmless. By small amounts I mean *less* than two drinks a day, preferably one drink. Try to imagine that heavy drinking is unattractive, that to be drunk or tight is unmanly and socially unacceptable because it suggests a loss of control. Such attitudes will help you to maintain your alcohol intake at a reasonable, harmless, perhaps even enjoyable level. If "What good is drinking if you cannot get drunk?" is your attitude, your risk of trouble is high.

If You Are in Trouble Now

If you have signs of symptomatic drinking, psychological dependence, frequent intoxication, the chances are that in the next few years you will face more trouble. You would probably do well to follow the tips for reduction of risk, although I am less hopeful that they will be as helpful to you as they will be for somebody who does not yet have a problem.

Symptomatic drinking and psychological dependence are signs of strong habits, probably as strong as or stronger than the eating habit of a person who is 30 per cent or more overweight. You probably need outside help in changing your drinking habit. And you can do it now, without hitting bottom. In other words, it is not necessary to wreck your life in order to change your drinking pattern; millions have done it. Why wait until the social punishment gets too great to bear?

10 / The Weed and Your Life

If You Smoke Cigarettes

Don't run away. I'm not going to harangue you about this most common of American habits. You will decide if you are going to quit, cut back, or keep on smoking. However, you have now read past the title of this chapter, which indicates a strong possibility that you want to quit or cut back. Somehow you believe there is a reason for your stopping. Maybe you realize that if you smoke cigarettes, your life is in danger.

As you probably know by now, a rational decision to change your behavior—regarding smoking or anything else—represents only the first step. Doing something about the decision is another story. Fortunately, behavioral scientists have studied cigarette-smoking intensively in the past few years. Although they have not come up with a foolproof method, they have some good ideas that can increase your chances of stopping or quitting if you want to. More than thirty million smokers have stopped. So it can be done.

Rather than give you all the data about disease and cigarette-smoking now, I will reverse the usual order of things to give you a chance to learn what there is to know about yourself, the kind of smoker you are, and smoking and health. Then I will try to show you what chance you have of stopping.

The best diagnostic tool is the Smoker's Self-Testing Kit, developed at the National Clearing House for Smoking and

Health by Dr. Daniel Horn and his colleagues. It is based on substantial evidence concerning almost six thousand smokers and nonsmokers. These tests have much in common with the alcohol tests in chapter 9, but Dr. Horn has refined them even beyond those.

Because Dr. Horn has done such a fine job, I have followed his self-testing kit closely, while interpolating data from his and other studies. The kit is a twelve-page pamphlet available for ten cents from the United States Government Printing Office as PHS Publication No. 1904. You may want additional copies for your friends, but all you need of it is here. There are four tests in the kit. After you take each test, score it. Then go on to the next test. After you have taken them all and figured your scores, read the explanation and the data. Do not cheat by trying to figure what the questions are getting at—not if you want an accurate self-appraisal. *Make sure you answer every question.*

Test No. 1: Do You Want to Change Your Smoking Habits?

For each statement below, circle the number that most accurately indicates how you feel.

	Completely Agree	Somewhat Agree	Somewhat Disagree	Completely Disagree
A. Cigarette-smoking might give me a serious illness.	4	3	2	1
B. My cigarette-smoking sets a bad example for others.	4	3	2	1
C. I find cigarette-smoking to be a messy habit.	4	3	2	1
D. Controlling my cigarette-smoking is a challenge to me.	4	3	2	1
E. Smoking causes shortness of breath.	4	3	2	1
F. If I quit smoking cigarettes it might influence others to stop.	4	3	2	1
G. Cigarettes cause damage to clothing and other personal property.	4	3	2	1

	Com- pletely Agree	Some- what Agree	Some- what Dis- agree	Com- pletely Dis- agree
H. Quitting smoking would show that I have willpower.	4	3	2	1
I. My cigarette-smoking will have a harmful effect on my health.	4	3	2	1
J. My cigarette-smoking influences others close to me to take up or continue smoking.	4	3	2	1
K. If I quit smoking, my sense of taste would improve.	4	3	2	1
L. I do not like the idea of feeling dependent on smoking.	4	3	2	1

SCORING TEST NO. 1. In the spaces below, enter the numbers you have circled in answer to the questions above. Put the number you circled in response to question A above the letter A, for question B above B, and so forth. Next, add the three numbers of each category *across* and enter the total above each word. A + E + I gives you the score for *Health.* B + F + J gives you the score for *Example,* et cetera. Your score can vary from 3 to 12. I will discuss its meaning later.

Totals

_____	+	_____	+	_____	=	_____
A		E		I		Health

_____	+	_____	+	_____	=	_____
B		F		J		Example

_____	+	_____	+	_____	=	_____
C		G		K		Esthetics

_____	+	_____	+	_____	=	_____
D		H		L		Mastery

Test No. 2: What Do You Think the Effects of Smoking Are?

Follow the instructions for the first test, circling the number that indicates how you feel about the statement.

	Strongly Agree	Mildly Agree	Mildly Dis- agree	Strongly Dis- agree
A. Cigarette-smoking is not nearly as dangerous as many other health hazards.	1	2	3	4
B. I don't smoke enough to get any of the diseases that ciga- rette-smoking is supposed to cause.	1	2	3	4
C. If a person has already smoked for many years, it probably won't do him much good to stop.	1	2	3	4
D. It would be hard for me to give up smoking cigarettes.	1	2	3	4
E. Cigarette-smoking is enough of a health hazard for some- thing to be done about it.	4	3	2	1
F. The kind of cigarette I smoke is much less likely than other kinds to give me any of the diseases that smoking is sup- posed to cause.	1	2	3	4
G. As soon as a person quits smoking cigarettes he begins to recover from much of the damage that smoking has caused.	4	3	2	1
H. It would be hard for me to cut down to half the number of cigarettes I now smoke.	1	2	3	4
I. The whole problem of ciga- rette-smoking and health is a very minor one.	1	2	3	4

	Strongly Agree	Mildly Agree	Mildly Disagree	Strongly Disagree
J. I haven't smoked long enough to worry about the diseases that cigarette-smoking is supposed to cause.	1	2	3	4
K. Quitting smoking helps a person live longer.	4	3	2	1
L. It would be difficult for me to make any substantial change in my smoking habits.	1	2	3	4

SCORING TEST NO. 2. Follow the same instructions as before, entering the number you have circled in answer to the question above the appropriate letter. Total the three scores across, as before.

				Totals
———— +	———— +	————	=	—————————
A	E	I		Importance
———— +	———— +	————	=	—————————
B	F	J		Personal Relevance
———— +	———— +	————	=	—————————
C	G	K		Value of Stopping
———— +	———— +	————	=	—————————
D	H	L		Capability of Stopping

Test No. 3: Why Do You Smoke?

This test includes statements made by various people to describe what they get out of smoking cigarettes. How often do you feel this way when smoking them?

	Always	Frequently	Occasionally	Seldom	Never
A. I smoke cigarettes in order to keep myself from slowing down.	5	4	3	2	1

	Always	Fre-quently	Occa-sionally	Sel-dom	Never
B. Handling a cigarette is part of the enjoyment of smoking it.	5	4	3	2	1
C. Smoking cigarettes is pleasant and relaxing.	5	4	3	2	1
D. I light up a cigarette when I feel angry about something.	5	4	3	2	1
E. When I run out of cigarettes I find it almost unbearable until I can get more.	5	4	3	2	1
F. I smoke automatically without even being aware of it.	5	4	3	2	1
G. I smoke to stimulate me, to perk myself up.	5	4	3	2	1
H. Part of the enjoyment of smoking a cigarette comes from the steps I take to light up.	5	4	3	2	1
I. I find cigarettes pleasurable.	5	4	3	2	1
J. When I feel uncomfortable or upset about something, I light up a cigarette.	5	4	3	2	1
K. When I am not smoking a cigarette, I am very much aware of the fact.	5	4	3	2	1
L. I light up a cigarette without realizing I still have one burning in the ashtray.	5	4	3	2	1
M. I smoke cigarettes to give me a "lift."	5	4	3	2	1

	Always	Fre-quently	Occa-sionally	Sel-dom	Never
N. When I smoke a cigarette, part of the enjoyment is watching the smoke as I exhale it.	5	4	3	2	1
O. I want a cigarette most when I am relaxed and comfortable.	5	4	3	2	1
P. When I feel blue or want to take my mind off cares and worries, I smoke.	5	4	3	2	1
Q. I get a real gnawing hunger for a cigarette when I haven't smoked for a while.	5	4	3	2	1
R. I've found a cigarette in my mouth and didn't remember putting it there.	5	4	3	2	1

SCORING TEST NO. 3. The instructions are the same as for those for scoring Nos. 1 and 2.

			Totals
A	+ G	+ M	= Stimulation
B	+ H	+ N	= Handling
C	+ I	+ O	= Pleasurable Relaxation
D	+ J	+ P	= Crutch: Tension Reduction
E	+ K	+ Q	= Craving: Psychological Addiction
F	+ L	+ R	= Habit

Test No. 4: Your Environment and Your Smoking

This test attempts to determine if the world around you will make it easier or harder for you to change your smoking habits. Again circle the appropriate numbers to indicate whether you feel the statements are true or false. Remember to answer every question.

	True or Mostly True	False or Mostly False
A. Doctors have decreased or stopped their smoking in the past ten years.	2	1
B. In recent years there seem to be more rules about where you are allowed to smoke.	2	1
C. Cigarette advertising makes smoking appear attractive to me.	1	2
D. Schools are trying to discourage children from smoking.	2	1
E. Doctors are trying to get their patients to stop smoking.	2	1
F. Someone has recently tried to persuade me to cut down or quit smoking cigarettes.	2	1
G. The widespread cigarette advertising makes it hard for me to quit smoking.	1	2
H. Both government and private health organizations are actively trying to discourage people from smoking.	2	1
I. A doctor has talked to me at least once about my smoking.	2	1
J. It seems as though an increasing number of people object to having someone smoke near them.	2	1
K. Some cigarette commercials on TV* make me feel like smoking.	1	2

* When Dr. Horn devised the test, television still carried cigarette commercials. Now it carries commercials only for cigars, little cigars, and pipe tobacco. Base your answer to K on how you remember cigarette commercials or on your reaction to the little-cigar commercials.

	True or Mostly True	*False or Mostly False*

L. Congressmen and other legislators are showing concern with smoking and health.   2   1

M. The people around you, particularly relatives, friends, office associates, may make it easier or more difficult for you to give up smoking by what they say or do. Would you say that they make giving it up or staying off cigarettes more difficult for you than it would be otherwise? (Circle the number to the left of the statement that best describes your situation.)

    3 They make it much more difficult than it would be otherwise.
    4 They make it somewhat more difficult.
    5 They make it somewhat easier.
    6 They make it much easier.

SCORING TEST NO. 4. Proceed as before, transferring the numbers and adding across for the separate totals.

				Totals
——— +	——— +	——— =	———	
A	E	I		Doctors
——— +	——— +	——— =	———	
B	F	J		General Climate
——— +	——— +	——— =	———	
C	G	K		Advertising Influence
——— +	——— +	——— =	———	
D	H	L		Key Group Influences
		——— =	———	
		M		Interpersonal Influences

Do not go on to the next section until you have finished all four tests. Go back and make sure you answered *every* question. Now you are ready to find out what kind of smoker you are and what your chances are of changing your smoking habit.

What It All Means

If I have given the impression in this book that it is easy to change habits of long standing, I did not mean to do so. Habits are hard to change, and for millions the most tenacious habit of all is cigarette-smoking. However, the range is very great. Many people find changing smoking habits relatively easy. In recent years such change has been helped along because the world has changed. There is no more television advertising of cigarettes; information about smoking and health has received wide distribution; warning labels have been printed on cigarettes; restrictions have sprung up about smoking on airplanes and in other public places.

In 1966, 56 per cent of Dr. Horn's smokers reported that they had *thought* of giving up smoking; by 1970 the figure had risen to 86 per cent. As for quitting, in 1966, 36 per cent of adults said they had tried to quit; in 1970, 57 per cent. In 1966, only 16 per cent of adults succeeded in staying off smoking for at least four weeks; by 1970 the figure had risen to 37 per cent. And finally, those who quit for at least one year: 7 per cent in 1966; 21 per cent in 1970. So things are improving, as you can see.

Changing America's Smoking Habits

	1966	1970
Thought of giving up	56%	86%
Tried to quit	36	57
Stayed off four weeks	16	37
Stayed off at least a year	7	21

If the per-capita smoking of cigarettes has not fallen off more dramatically than this study suggests, it is because teen-agers are taking up smoking in greater numbers than before. In two years, between 1968 and 1970, the number of regular smokers among seventeen- and eighteen-year-old boys increased by 20 per cent; the same was true for girls in that age group. In 1972, there were indications that the teen-age trend might be leveling off.

The Horn study and others indicate clearly that a growing awareness of the habit as a health risk will lead to a tendency to discontinue the habit. Eighty-four per cent of teen-agers said they know that cigarette-smoking is harmful to health, and more than half of them said they won't be smoking five years from the time they were interviewed.

INTERPRETING TEST NO. 1. Do you believe strongly enough that smoking is harmful to health? If your score on the *health* factor is 6 or lower, then you just do not know enough of the facts about smoking.

If you scored 9 or above on the *example* factor, it means that you are quite concerned with the effect your smoking has on others. You believe you have an impact on the people around you. This high sense of responsibility is enough to induce some people to stop smoking. Parents often stop because they do not want to set a "bad" example for their children. If parents smoke, there is a high probability of their children smoking. So if you score high, you are ripe for quitting.

If you scored low, 6 or less, then you do not have an image of yourself as important in other people's lives. If you are married, you probably do not think that your smoking has any real impact on your spouse. Some of your fellow workers may be having a hard time stopping because you are puffing away all around them. If you try to realize that each of us—you included—has an effect on the people around us, then maybe you can increase this score by just watching people react to your smoking.

I score very high on the *esthetic* factor, because I believe that cigarette-smoking is a messy habit. When my wife and I have company, the one thing we dread is cleaning the ashtrays, and, alas, sometimes the burns in our furniture. If you, too, have a score of 9 or higher, you are simply fed up with the bad esthetics of smoking—the smell of stale smoke on clothes, the stains on your fingers and teeth, and the bad breath. A high score means you may be ready to give up smoking on this basis alone.

If you scored low—6 or less—you might think about the fact that cigarette-smoking *is* a messy business. Look at your fingers. Are they stained yellow? Think about what other people might say about that . . . or your teeth . . . hard to keep them white? How about the furniture burns? Has someone turned away from you when you tried to kiss them? Maybe it's the tobacco smell.

A score of 9 or above in *mastery* means that you are troubled by the fact that cigarettes have made you a slave, that you cannot seem to quit. A lot of people are bothered this way: they do not want to give up being human, that is, having control over their lives. And yet here they are trapped by a three-inch cylinder filled with a noxious weed. If you scored low, then you do not seem to mind that you cannot get rid of the habit, and that will go against your being able to quit.

A score above 9 on any factor—*health, example, esthetics, mastery*—may be enough to induce you to want to stop now. The strongest reason for most people is health. So if your health score is low, it is a good idea to take a look at how you did on Test No. 2. Incidentally, even if you scored low on all four parts of Test No. 1, I hope that you may still find elsewhere in this chapter a way of increasing your willingness to try to change your cigarette habit.

INTERPRETING TEST NO. 2. This test goes a little deeper than Test No. 1 by trying to give you some idea of your attitudes on smoking and your chances of quitting. Those attitudes can be derived from scoring yourself on the *importance* of the risk of smoking to health, the *relevance* of that risk to you (do *you* see it as important for you?), the *value* to be gained from stopping, and the *capability*, as you see it, that you have for stopping.

A low score—6 or less—on *importance* means that you do not think that cigarette-smoking produces dangerous effects on human beings. This is a popular belief among smokers, for it serves to rationalize their habit. After all, what reasonable person would continue a habit if there were a high risk attached to it? So the way to handle it is simply to minimize that risk intellectually rather than stop smoking.

Much of the resistance to the idea that cigarette-smoking causes death and disability is a result of the propaganda of the cigarette makers. It is not difficult to understand their enthusiasm: they are trying to protect a multibillion-dollar business. They have made statistics the villain, claiming that there is no "real" evidence linking cigarette-smoking to lung cancer, heart disease, or emphysema. What they are ignoring, however, is the fact that statistics have been the basis for every major public-health advance and have saved literally millions of lives. You can go back to the cholera epidemics of the nineteenth century, before the germ theory, and find that a statistical study implicated a contaminated water well; the effectiveness of the polio vaccine was demonstrated with statistics; and statistics now reveal the punishing power of our saturated-fats diet.

Almost fifty years ago, a statistical study conducted by Dr. Raymond Pearl of Johns Hopkins University showed that men who smoked cigarettes were dying twice as fast as those who did not. Since then there have been at least seven major studies, involving more than a million men, that show clearly that smokers die faster than nonsmokers.

A twenty-five-year-old man who smokes two packs of cigarettes a day can expect to have eight years chopped off his life expectancy. Figures for women are not yet obtainable, because women have not been smoking in large enough numbers for a long enough time. However, preliminary data suggests that early death will hold among women smokers, although not as strongly.

The statistics show that the average man who smokes has ten times more chances of contracting lung cancer than the nonsmoker. The two-pack-a-day man has sixty-four times more chances.

But even more important than lung cancer is coronary artery disease, because so many more men die of this disease than of lung cancer. Among American men who smoke, lung cancer accounts for only 13 per cent of the extra risk of death; coronary disease, 51 per cent. Suppose in a given year there are 1,000 male smokers who die. In a group of nonsmokers of the same number, statistics show that only 600 die. Of the 400 excess deaths, only 52 are attributed to lung cancer—and more than 200 to coronary disease. Thus the greater problem generated by cigarette-smoking is heart disease, not lung cancer—although of course that is not to be overlooked.

There are many who say, "So what? So I die a few years earlier. At least I will have enjoyed my life." That attitude would be okay if it were based on fact. But recent studies suggest that smokers who die young are generally sicker than those who die later. The United States Public Health Service estimates that smokers are generally sicker than nonsmokers. They spend more time ill in bed, lose more days at work, and have to restrict their activity more than nonsmokers. In a year the illness of smokers as compared with that of nonsmokers accounted for an extra 88,000,000 days spent in bed, 77,000,000 working days lost, and

306,000,000 days of restricted activity. For men between the ages of forty-five and sixty-four, the extra illness represented almost a third of all the days of disability in that age group.

It is pretty clear that you pay for your cigarette-smoking with early death and more illness. So if your score on *importance* in Test No. 2 was low, you should reconsider your position in the light of the evidence. More than that, even if you are not a heavy—two-pack—smoker, a small number of cigarettes a day carries a freight of harm. Many people ask, "Doesn't air pollution have a bigger effect than cigarettes?" No. While it is difficult to prove any health effects from air pollution, it is easy to prove that air pollution is a trivial worry compared with the impact of smoking even one pack of cigarettes a day, much less two. Aside from the cancer-provoking chemicals that cigarettes certainly contain, there is so much carbon monoxide in the smoke stream that it would signal a national emergency if it were in the air in proportionate amounts. Carbon monoxide in cigarettes is believed by many to be the agent that triggers heart attacks, because it cuts down the oxygen supply in the blood.

A low score on *personal relevance* indicates that you probably have the soldier-on-the-battlefield syndrome: the bullet is for somebody else—and if it *is* for you, nothing can stop it. You will be less willing to try to stop smoking. For example, you probably tend *not* to believe that a small number of cigarettes can hurt you; yet research indicates that even half a pack a day begins to reduce your lung capacity after a few years. Emphysema—in which the victim feels as though he is drowning; it can go on for years before it kills him—can be triggered by modest amounts of smoking.

If your score is 6 or less, you just do not have the facts . . . and you are in a vulnerable position.

Do you believe that you have smoked so long that it is too late, you already have the disease? A score below 6 on the *value of stopping* indicates that you hold this belief. Well, you are wrong. Research studies show quite clearly that the risk of heart disease, lung cancer, and death decline year by year after you stop smoking. You never quite catch up to the nonsmokers if you have been smoking a couple of packs a day, but after about five years your risk has dropped 20 per cent; after ten years it is down 30 per cent. If you smoke only a pack a day or less, your risk of death or disease after ten years is almost that of the nonsmoker.

A low score in *capability of stopping* suggests that you have no confidence in your ability to overcome your smoking habit; perhaps you have failed several times. But you should take heart from the fact that it is not impossible to stop. Thirty million Americans *have quit;* if they can, you can. More impressive, perhaps, is the fact that one hundred thousand doctors have stopped smoking, representing half the doctors who ever smoked. That emphasizes one of the most important reasons for quitting: the connection between disease and smoking.

ARE YOU READY? If you scored high on the first two tests, you are ready to quit smoking or at least to cut back dramatically. All you have to do is decide. Remember, there are different kinds of smokers. In your past attempts to stop, perhaps you used the wrong tactics for the kind of smoker you are. If you decide to try, the next sections will help you figure out a plan of attack.

If you scored low on both tests, you are not ready to try. Perhaps at this point you should try some behavior-modification techniques. First, go back and see where your scores are weak. If it is in *health*, try rereading the sections on evidence connecting cigarette smoking and disease. Then you can use the thought-punishment idea: imagine yourself with lung cancer . . . dying of a heart attack . . . unable to breathe with emphysema. If you can make yourself believe that these things can happen to you, then you may be able to increase your motivation to quit.

Look over each score and go back to the statements, reviewing your feelings about them. Is it that you do not really think cigarette-smoking is messy? Think of all the places you've been where cigarettes are on the floor, on the table, even in your coffee cup! Is it that you do not believe you set an example for anybody? You do. Each of us does. Think of the people around you, the smokers and nonsmokers; they are in some way influenced by you.

INTERPRETING TEST NO. 3. Everybody knows that for many smokers nicotine provides a "lift." But not everybody responds to the drug in the same way. In trying to understand the nature of the reward in cigarette smoking, Dr. Silvan S. Tomkins, professor of psychology at Rutgers University, hit upon a theory about why people smoke: in some way smoking helps them manage their emotions.

All of us sometimes feel depressed or tired or worried. How do we manage those emotions? Some of us talk to people. Some grin and bear it. Others take pills or have a drink. Another answer is a cigarette. But for many, what begins as a quick, cheap way of dealing with an emotional upset passes on to psychological dependence or to pure, unthinking habit. When Dr. Horn conducted his national surveys, the smokers seemed to fall into the theoretical categories that Dr. Tomkins had established. Knowing in which group you belong can help you quit or change your smoking behavior.

Of the six categories, the first three are positive feelings that people get from smoking: *stimulation,* the "lift" that people report when they smoke; the physical satisfaction of *handling* the cigarette; the *pleasurable relaxation* many smokers get from lighting up, particularly after a meal, say, or while reading a good book or having a good conversation. Test No. 3 measures these factors.

Stimulation. If you scored 11 or above, the stimulation you get from cigarettes is important to you—it keeps you going through a tedious job or wakes you up in the morning or helps you to organize yourself. The problem in giving up smoking is to find a substitute for that stimulation. Unfortunately, many smokers turn to amphetamines to pep them up. But what you need are safe substitutes. For waking up in the morning, you can follow the suggestions in the chapter on sleep. For example, when you set the alarm clock have a Thermos of orange juice, coffee, or tea at the bedside and reward yourself for putting your feet on the floor by taking a sip of the liquid.

In the chapter on work habits, I describe some substitutes for cigarette-smoking in helping you to get through a tedious job. Essentially, you set up the work in a way that provides for ongoing rewards when you complete small portions of the job. Again, a sip of a cold or hot (noncaloric) drink will provide enough stimulation to keep you going. Dr. Horn suggests a brisk walk for stimulation. I think a cold shower helps; even moderate exercise will do it.

People in this category need not stop smoking all at once; they may be able to taper off if they can find *safe* substitutes for the stimulation that cigarettes give them. However, it is better to stop smoking all at once, and use the substitutes to keep you from starting again.

Handling. If you scored high—11 or above—you get more pleasure out of the whole ritual of handling the cigarette than out of smoking itself. You like to take the cigarette out of its package, tap it, smooth it, light it, and watch the smoke. In this case, you ought to find something else to play with to keep your hands busy: a pen, pencil, piece of jewelry. How about doodling? Dr. Horn suggests plastic cigarettes, maybe even a real one if you can trust yourself not to light it. You can also roll two steel ball bearings together in your hand, as Captain Queeg did in *The Caine Mutiny* (though for a different reason).

Pleasurable Relaxation. Dr. Horn points out that it is not always apparent whether a person smokes for a pleasant sensation or to keep from feeling bad. Thus the answers to this group (C, I, O) can easily overlap with those for the next category (*Crutch: Tension Reduction*). In fact, many smokers score high—11 or better —in both.

But if you are the kind of smoker who gets simple satisfaction out of smoking, then it is easy to substitute other satisfying activities and not miss cigarettes. You must be careful not to turn to eating or drinking; either one can get you into other kinds of trouble. Meeting with friends, talking on the telephone, and other social activities are good substitutes. So are going to the movies, reading, watching television, and playing games. Some people have taken up exercise as a substitute for smoking and it works perfectly well.

Crutch: Tension Reduction. The people in this category show some similarity, in my view, to those individuals who show a high risk for getting into trouble over alcohol—they use a drug to control negative feelings.

Smokers who score high—11 or above—use the cigarette as a tranquilizing, psychic crutch in moments of stress. They may find it easy to quit when things are going well. But the moment there is trouble, they reach for a cigarette. That is when the substitute should be ready and practiced.

One good one—which also works for avoiding high-calorie foods—is to use the power of thought punishments to deter your taking a cigarette. At the moment the signal for the start of smoking behavior appears, evoke a scene that is sufficiently terrible so that you do not reach for or accept a cigarette: your lungs are coated with soot . . . you are coughing up blood . . . you have a cancer as big as a basketball growing in your chest. As soon as the craving for a cigarette stops, stop the thought immediately by shouting to yourself, Stop! Then turn to some substitute activity.

Craving: Psychological Addiction. A smoker who scored 11 or above in this category has all the earmarks of the person who is psychologically dependent on alcohol. He begins to miss his cigarette—just as the alcohol-dependent person misses alcohol—the minute he puts it out. The longer he goes without smoking, the more he misses it. Such smokers are among those who find quitting extremely difficult. Tapering off does no good; the moment they light another cigarette, the addiction reasserts itself. So the advice is: cold turkey. Stop all at once. Grin and bear it.

Dr. Horn suggests that it may be helpful to smoke excessively for a day or two to spoil the taste of cigarettes and then to isolate yourself completely from them. That means throwing out all unused packs, sitting in the no-smoking areas of trains and lounges, perhaps even taking a trip to an isolated location where no cigarettes are available.

Behavior-modification techniques can help. Once you recognize the stimulus that sets off the craving, you can intervene to prevent yourself from taking a cigarette—just as an eater prevents himself from taking that extra helping. Remember that you have to have a thought punishment powerful enough to offset the craving. (Dr. Horn says that giving up cigarettes may be so difficult and cause so much pain that the smoker who does quit will find it easier to stay off than to go through all the pain of quitting again.)

Substitute activities will help. Be wary of choosing eating or drinking or pills—you are the type who could easily become dependent on them.

Habit. For those of you who score 11 or higher in this category, smoking has become like tying your shoelaces: you no longer even know you are doing it. It is a tic, a pure physical habit with practically no psychological overtones. You no longer even enjoy cigarettes. You just light them up and let them go.

Fortunately, such habits are easy to change. It requires a careful analysis of the steps you go through to smoke. And if you change the steps, you can back off the habit. For example, if you put your cigarettes in a different pocket, tie the pack up with rubber bands, or even keep an empty pack in your pocket, you will end up smoking fewer cigarettes.

Dr. Horn suggests that the key to success is to become aware of each cigarette that you smoke and to ask yourself: "Do I really want this cigarette?" That breaks up the chain of behavior and you will find yourself wanting cigarettes less and less frequently.

You can turn off any step of the behavior chain with thought punishments and thus prevent yourself from going to the next step. You can also paint a bitter-tasting fluid, such as the kind used for getting children to stop biting their nails, on the ends of a *random* number of cigarettes in the pack. When you put one of those cigarettes in your mouth unthinkingly, the bitter taste will remind you to stop.

If you scored low (below 7) on all six categories, you probably do not smoke much or have not been smoking for long. In either case it should be easy for you to quit—and you now have the motivation gained from understanding the unhealthy aspects of smoking.

If you scored high on two or more factors, you may have to use multiple strategies to counteract each of the kinds of pleasure (reward) that smoking gives you. A high score on both *Crutch: Tension Relaxation* and *Craving: Psychological Addiction* makes for a particularly tough combination. Dr. Horn suggests changing your pattern for a few months by smoking low-tar-and-nicotine cigarettes, inhaling less often and less deeply, while at the same time cutting down the number of cigarettes. Then the leap to cold turkey won't be quite so devastating.

INTERPRETING TEST NO. 4. In addition to your own behavior during the period when you are trying to quit, there may be factors in your environment that need managing. Remember, the idea is to cut down on smoking stimuli wherever they occur in your life.

A score not lower than 5 or 6 on the *Doctors* factor means you have confidence in your doctor; he can be helpful in motivating you to stop smoking. However, I do not suggest that you ask him for pills to help you over your nervousness during the quitting period. (Incidentally, hypnosis works for some people, but I have seen no evidence that it works any better than the techniques outlined by Dr. Horn.)

A low score—3 or 4 or less—on *General Climate* indicates that you find your living and working environments not congenial to a quitting program. You may have to try associating, for a few months, anyway, with nonsmokers, going to places where smoking is prohibited (the nonsmoking sections of moviehouses), asking people to stop smoking in your presence, asking them not to offer you cigarettes, et cetera.

Since television no longer carries cigarette commercials, the *Advertising Influence* may not be a big problem for you. A score of 3 or 4 or lower dictates that you would be strongly influenced by such commercials to light up—so watch out for the little-cigar, cigar, and pipe commercials. When they come on, leave the room. Get a drink of water.

In *Key Group Influences,* a score of not lower than 5 or 6 suggests that you are aware of the fact that most health agencies, the Federal Government, school agencies, and doctors are now strongly against cigarette-smoking. There is no real controversy in the scientific community, except for a few individuals. If you have a low score, you did not realize that in this country cigarette-smoking is no longer regarded as a minor vice, but a major health problem.

Your family and friends can have a great deal of influence on your behavior. An un-co-operative spouse, for instance, can be a major factor in the breakdown of a behavior-change program, be it an anticholesterol diet or a no-smoking regime. A score of not higher than 3 or 4 on *Interpersonal Influences* means you are vulnerable to just such problems. If you can get your spouse to quit while you are trying to, you will be way ahead of the game.

The Decision

Cigarette-smoking is a learned habit arrived at, as Dr. Horn has shown, by different routes for different people. Each smoker derives a different habit-reinforcing reward, which he can use to stop smoking. The steps are simple:

1. Find out if you are sufficiently motivated to stop (Test Nos. 1 and 2).

2. Find out what type of smoker you are (Test No. 3).

3. Devise a suitable strategy, using behavior-modification techniques to help you change your patterns.

4. In case of failure, start all over again.

Since motivation to stop is so important and depends so much on what you know about smoking, you should reread this chapter, and also read anything else that points out the dangers of smoking in a reasonable way. When I was science editor at the New York *Herald Tribune,* a series of associates who came my way were smokers. My strategy in getting them to stop was merely to assign them to any and all cigarette stories. The act of researching and writing the articles was enough to make all of them quit (although one did resume smoking later). That is the same force that was at work with the one hundred thousand doctors who quit: they knew more about disease and were in a position to read more about smoking and health.

That is the program, the best science has to offer. It is not magic. It does take effort . . . but millions have succeeded. So can you. The question: Do you want to?

11 / Sex and Behavior

What Do You Want?

Nobody wants a bad sex life; a substantial number of people—so some studies show—want no sex life; but the overwhelming majority—the exact figure is unknown—want a good sex life. Of course, "good" and "bad" mean different things to different people, even within the same marriage or relationship.

Discussion of this complex human behavior is not so difficult as it might at first seem. Researchers have simplified the problem by establishing four factors that are present in every sex life: frequency of sexual behavior; degree of intensity; the nature, or mood; the duration. There is no "perfect" record implicit in any of these. They simply provide a handy subject guide for establishing the pattern of a particular person's sexual life. The question of whether or not that pattern is satisfactory is answerable only by each of us, according to our own preferences and standards.

The first is the apparently simple matter of establishing how many times a day, a week, a month or year we perform some kind of sexual act, be it intercourse, masturbation, petting, or whatever. Thirty years ago, Dr. Alfred C. Kinsey and his associates interviewed several thousand Americans on their sexual habits and discovered that the frequency range varied from zero per month to several times a day. Inevitably, in the aftermath of this rather sensational study, many people compared their own frequency average with that established by Kinsey's findings, and in so doing overemphasized the importance of frequency. If they fell below the average activity, they immediately assumed they were inadequate; above the average meant either that they were in the realm of sexual champions or were slightly "sex mad." What they failed to grasp is that frequency is only part of the whole picture. I cannot emphasize enough that if you think *only* of the number of times you have sex, you are missing out on the other benefits of a good sex life.

Intensity, the second factor, is the degree of sensation during the sex act. Contrary to what you may have read or heard, the physical sensations of sex vary not only from person to person, but from time to time in the same person. Part of the popular notion about intercourse is that there should be fireworks every time; experiencing only mildly pleasant feelings suggests to many people, wrongly, a failure in some sense. For many, the whole experience of the sex act is concentrated toward achieving an orgasm. But here again it is a matter of understanding the fact that different people react differently during sex; the standards are always personal. One's own experiences should not be compared with another's. Although the idea of being a championship tennis player is exciting, consider that a good game of tennis is quite satisfying. Similarly with sex: there is no need to consider it a championship athletic performance geared exclusively to achieving an orgasm. There are many other possible levels of enjoyment.

What is an orgasm? If you have ever had one, you probably know exactly what it is; if you are not sure you have had one, you probably haven't. Many women experience orgasm but are not aware that that is what it is called. In essence, an orgasm is an intense tingling and tension-releasing feeling concentrated in the pelvic region and often spreading out to affect the entire body.

Men generally have one orgasm at a time, which is separated from the next by a period during which they are unable to achieve orgasm, even if they make an extra effort. But they can still feel sexual arousal—they can be "turned on" sexually. By the time they reach adulthood, most men have experienced orgasm one way or another, although there are some men who never achieve it. On the other hand, women are capable of experiencing multiple orgasms, one right after another. However, many women —perhaps even one-third—never experience it.

The third factor, the nature of the sex act, is the mood evoked. A spontaneous feeling of tenderness toward the sexual partner may be what is important or desirable for one person. For another, the daydreams or fantasies that accompany sexual arousal through masturbation represent "good" sex. Many people regard sex as a purely physical release; the mood, if any, is irrelevant. Others are quite content to experience a sense of physical and emotional closeness with another person without orgasmic release.

The nature of the act—the mood evoked—makes sex for human beings profoundly different from the sex acts of animals. Most women seem to derive the most pleasure from sex when it is accompanied by emotional feelings of attachment, of love. Most men want the same thing; but generally, they find such mood aspects less important. However, it should be pointed out that too much has been made of the difference between men and women on this point. What stands out is that if the mood is elevated by feelings of love, intimacy, caring, and attachment, sex is considered better by both men and women.

Finally, there is duration. How long does the sex act take? Two minutes, fifteen minutes, an hour? Obviously, there can be no set time period. An hour of sexual effort can have no rewards at all. On the other hand, a person who seeks only physical release may find two minutes quite adequate.

Frequency, intensity, nature, and duration—FIND. Each of these varies enormously from person to person. There is no absolute, ideal combination. Sex behavior depends on an individual's biology, upbringing, early sex experience, partner—or lack of one—imagination, and know-how. It also depends, as does the person's overall feeling about sex, on what you want.

What do you want? Do you want sex more often? Or do you want better sex? Or do you want your sexual act to last longer each time? The gap between what you want and what you do represents the degree to which you are dissatisfied with your current sex life. Perhaps you have never considered whether you were dissatisfied or, if you were, never expressed the fact explicitly. Perhaps you have had vague feelings of unhappiness about your sex life but have not known how to pinpoint the sources of the difficulties. If you understand how and why you are dissatisfied, you might be able to do something about it—using reward/ punishment theory.

Satisfied or Dissatisfied?

At one time, it was a common conception that the only way in which most people achieved sexual release was through hetero-sexual intercourse between husband and wife in the face-to-face position with the man on top. Masturbation was for little boys. Prostitutes were supposed to be visited only by single men. And then there were the writings of Richard Krafft-Ebing that detailed the activities of the "weirdos." Homosexuality was considered a rare aberration.

Scientific scrutiny has in the recent past provided us with a somewhat broader view. Dr. Kinsey showed that masturbation is quite common among older, married males; that sexual inter-course involves not only a variety of positions, but such acts as oral-genital contact and even anal intercourse; that one man in five has performed a homosexual act and perhaps one woman in ten has; that a small percentage of men has had sexual contact with animals.

Such a broad range of possibilities precludes my providing you with a simple recipe for curing your dissatisfactions. What I can do is present some scientific findings; then it will be up to you to apply them to your particular situation. For example, much of what I report will deal with male-female sexuality. Those who prefer homosexual activity will be able to apply the findings to their own situation, according to their understanding of the differences between heterosexual and homosexual activity.

Perhaps one thing that many people with problems fail to realize is that the health of a relationship depends on both sexual satisfaction and agreeable personal feelings. If the feelings be-tween two people are bad—negative in some way—then no matter how good the sex may be, the relationship is likely to be unsatis-factory. On the other hand, if the sex is unsatisfactory, the rela-tionship is bound to suffer, no matter how good the other feelings are. There are many couples who live sexless lives. I cite this not as a goal, but in order to emphasize the variety of human rela-tionships.

You may be dissatisfied about the nature of the sexual acts your partner desires. Suppose everything you learned about sex has convinced you that sexual intercourse with the woman on her back and the man on top facing her is the only natural, moral way of sex. If your mate learned and yearns for other ways, there will be deep mutual dissatisfaction if you permit only your way.

No matter what your particular difficulty may be, there can be an improvement if the dissatisfaction is made explicit. If you understand where the gaps are, you can take steps to change your behavior, using techniques now being rapidly developed.

Assessing Your Sex Behavior

To close the existing gaps, start by taking some measure of your satisfactions and dissatisfactions and those of your mate. Dr. Joseph LoPiccolo, who has developed a sexual-growth program at the University of Oregon, Eugene, devised an inventory of sexual behavior and desires that helps him to help those in need. He has found that the inventory can be a useful guide in changing sex behavior. The test covers seventeen types of sexual activity, for each of which there are six questions. Dr. LoPiccolo does not want his inventory used by nonprofessionals, so I cannot reproduce it here. However, using the same idea, I have selected, out of the vast number of possibilities, eleven sexual acts that form the basis of a sex-behavior assessment. A few of them will be embarrassing to some of you and interesting to others, but your response, whatever it is, will help you understand your own sexuality. An ideal way of improving your sexual behavior, if that is what you want, is for both you and your partner to do assessments—provided, of course, that you do not make it an occasion for accusation and recrimination. Agree in advance that you are going to use the results only to close the gaps.

The sex-behavior assessment that follows is not meant to measure sexual athletic ability. Rather, it attempts to measure the difference between what you do and what you want. So don't cheat by bragging that you do more than you actually do; don't play the sophisticate by indicating things that you do not want simply because you think your partner will want them. If you want to help yourself, answer as truthfully as you can.

Notice that there are eleven sexual acts listed, each with categories showing frequency or duration. Circle the number beside the category that best represents your estimate of how often you do that particular act, how often you want to do it, and how often you think your partner wants to. If your partner is also doing an assessment, he or she should write the circled number on a separate sheet of paper. Compare your scores later, after you have taken the test.

Sex-Behavior Assessment

	Activity occurs	*You want activity to occur*	*You think your partner wants activity*
Kissing and caressing partner			
Daily	4	4	4
Three times weekly	3	3	3
Weekly	2	2	2
Less than weekly	1	1	1
You say endearing words during sex play and intercourse			
Almost always	4	4	4
More than half the time	3	3	3
Less than half the time	2	2	2
Almost never	1	1	1
Your partner says endearing words to you during sex play and intercourse			
Almost always	4	4	4
More than half the time	3	3	3
Less than half the time	2	2	2
Almost never	1	1	1
Sex play and intercourse usually lasts*			
Less than five minutes	1	1	1
Five to fifteen minutes	2	2	2
Fifteen to thirty minutes	3	3	3
More than half an hour	4	4	4

* For columns 1, 2, and 3, read: sex play and sexual intercourse usually lasts, you want sex play and sexual intercourse to last, and you think your partner wants them to last, respectively.

	Activity occurs	You want activity to occur	You think your partner wants activity
Man fondles woman's breast			
Daily	4	4	4
Three times weekly	3	3	3
Weekly	2	2	2
Less than weekly	1	1	1
Man strokes woman's genital area			
Daily	4	4	4
Three times weekly	3	3	3
Weekly	2	2	2
Less than weekly	1	1	1
Woman strokes man's genitals			
Daily	4	4	4
Three times weekly	3	3	3
Weekly	2	2	2
Less than weekly	1	1	1
Sexual intercourse with or without orgasm			
Daily	4	4	4
Three times weekly	3	3	3
Weekly	2	2	2
Less than weekly	1	1	1
Sexual intercourse with orgasm			
Daily	4	4	4
Three times weekly	3	3	3
Weekly	2	2	2
Less than weekly	1	1	1
Woman kisses or touches man's genitals with her mouth			
Daily	4	4	4
Three times weekly	3	3	3
Weekly	2	2	2
Less than weekly	1	1	1

	Activity occurs	You want activity to occur	You think your partner wants activity
Man kisses or touches woman's genitals with his mouth			
Daily	4	4	4
Three times weekly	3	3	3
Weekly	2	2	2
Less than weekly	1	1	1

Scoring Your Sex-Behavior Assessment

1. Activity (add your circled numbers in column 1) —— (1)
2. Desire (add your circled numbers in column 2) —— (2)
3. Estimate of partner's desire (add your circled numbers in column 3) —— (3)
4. Partner's activity (add your partner's circled numbers in column 1) —— (4)
5. Partner's desire (add partner's circled numbers in column 2) —— (5)
6. Partner's estimate of your desire (add partner's circled numbers in column 3) —— (6)

A. Personal satisfaction/dissatisfaction
   (subtract line 2 from line 1 above) —— (A)
B. Partner's satisfaction/dissatisfaction
   (subtract line 5 from line 4 above) —— (B)
C. Desire difference
   (subtract line 5 from line 2 above) —— (C)
D. Your reading of partner's desires
   (subtract line 5 from line 3 above) —— (D)
E. Partner's reading of your desires
   (subtract line 2 from line 6 above) —— (E)
F. Activity gap
   (subtract line 4 from line 1 above) —— (F)

Note: Some of the subtractions will produce minus numbers. For example, suppose your activity score (1) is 21 and your desire score (2) is 38. Simply subtract 21 from 38 and put a minus sign in front of the answer (−17).

Interpreting the Scores

Ignore scores 1 through 6. They are only numbers to help you get to the real issues as revealed by scores A through F. Different people have different drives and background that will yield different scores. Thus there is no absolutely "good" activity score. What you really want is an estimate of the differences between activity and desire, between your desires and your partner's, between what you think your partner wants and what your partner actually wants. If your partner did not do the assessment, then only the personal satisfaction/dissatisfaction score can be determined. Of the fifteen different scores that can be calculated from the Sex-Behavior Assessment, I have selected only six as being relevant for changing your behavior.

A. PERSONAL SATISFACTION/DISSATISFACTION. This number measures the gap between your sex activity and your desire. A minus score means you are dissatisfied; you want more sex than you are having. A zero score or one close to zero means that you are as active as you desire. A positive or plus score means you are involved in more sex activity than you really want.

Score	Comment
−5 to +5	You are well satisfied. Your sex needs pretty well match your sex activity.
−5 to −10	You are moderately dissatisfied. You want more sex activity than you are now having.
below −10	You are strongly dissatisfied and want much more sex activity than you are now having. You must proceed carefully with your partner in discussing this gap.
below −25	You have serious sexual dissatisfactions—to the point where you may need special help.
+5 to +10	You are moderately dissatisfied because too much sexual demand is being made upon you.
above +10	You are strongly dissatisfied; the demands on you go beyond your desire.
above +25	Your partner is making very strong sex demands on you that go beyond your desire; there may be serious problems between you.

As you notice, each score measures the difference between what you do and what you want. However, even with a low-difference score there may still be gaps that are hidden by the method of scoring. Thus a large positive gap on one item may cover a large negative gap on another. For example, suppose you are a woman who wants sexual intercourse, with or without orgasm, once a week, but you are having it daily. On the other hand, you want your partner to say endearing words to you during intercourse almost always and he never says them. The two items would score as follows:

	Activity occurs	*You want activity*
Intercourse	4	2
Endearing words	1	4
Totals	5	6
Difference score: −1		

Although the difference score is only −1, there are big gaps between your desires and your activity on the two items. Therefore, it is a good idea to look at individual items for further clues to dissatisfactions. Indeed, you will learn more about your partner and yourself if you look at individual differences rather than take the numerical scores too seriously. In fact, there is little objective evidence that gives validity to the scores—they are only indicators.

B. PARTNER'S SATISFACTION/DISSATISFACTION. This is to be interpreted exactly like A. It is a good idea to look over the items together. However, be cautious; you or your partner may have strong feelings about particular items.

C. DESIRE DIFFERENCE. The interpretation is similar to that of the A and B scores. A figure close to zero indicates that the partners have similar sex-desire levels, although they may be far apart on special items. A minus score for you indicates that your partner's sex desires are stronger than yours; a plus score indicates that your sex needs are more urgent. The score number has about the same meaning as those of A and B. To close the gap the desire of the lower-scoring partner could be raised. Logically, the desire of the more needful partner could be lessened, but that might more easily lead to difficulty in the relationship.

D AND E. READING EACH OTHER'S DESIRES. Because sex is such a taboo subject, even between married people, the chances are that neither you nor your partner really understands what it is each of you wants in sex. Silent ignorance prevails. If these scores are zero or close to it, you read each other well. The higher the scores, the greater the misunderstanding. Perhaps you think your partner wants sexual intercourse daily; it turns out your partner is satisfied with three times a week. You find out your partner thinks you want to hear endearing words during intercourse; you really want none of it. The assessment can provide a helpful launch pad for sexual communication, one of the most vital, and usually missing, ingredients in improving the frequency, intensity, nature, and duration of sexual activity. Again, look at individual items rather than the overall score.

F. ACTIVITY GAP. This score reveals to what degree you and your partner differ on the "facts" about your sex life. Dr. Kinsey discovered that often the sexual-intercourse frequency reported to him by one marriage partner differed from that of the other. Wives said they were having more sexual intercourse with their husbands than their husbands said they were having. A low score means you and your partner agree on the facts. A high score means disagreement—one of you believes more is happening than actually occurs, the other believes less is happening. There is an easy way to resolve such differences. You keep track of what you are doing, a method, as we shall see, that has more important implications than merely settling an argument.

What to Do?

If you have serious, longstanding sex problems, you may be beyond the help of this book. If you are a woman who has never had an orgasm during sexual intercourse or a man who cannot control his ejaculations, you may be able to solve the problem by following some of the suggestions below. But if the problems are locked-in habits, you may need special guidance and training. Just such help has been devised by Dr. William H. Masters and Mrs. Virginia E. Johnson, of the Reproductive Biology Research Foundation in St. Louis, Missouri. They have described their methods in a book called *Human Sexual Inadequacy. Understanding Human Sexual Inadequacy,* by Fred Belliveau and Lin Richter, might also be helpful. It is not so technical as the former, is easier to read, and provides many good ideas for the sexually unhappy. You might also be able to take advantage of the special sex-treatment centers that have begun to spring up in many different cities.

But if you feel that your sex problems place you in a somewhat more average category, you can do much on your own to solve them, provided you want to do so. Now that you have made an assessment—by no means exhaustive—of your sex behavior, you are in a position to do something about the gaps revealed. The benefits abound. A good sex life can mean living longer (there is evidence that married people outlive unmarried) and enjoying better health. To perform sexually, you have to be in good physical condition. Sex activity provides a positive reward for keeping in good shape by exercise, diet, and avoidance of drinking and smoking. Alcohol, barbiturates, and the opiates definitely decrease sexual competence. I strongly believe that if you want to convince a person to exercise regularly and keep slim, suggest to him that one of the greatest benefits will be a luxurious sexual existence. Many physicians have observed the slimming down of middle-aged men who have taken young sex partners. The waning of sexual activity with age may be attributed more to the decline of physical vigor and the onset of overweight than to depression of the sexual function per se. Figures indicate that 63 per cent of men over the age of fifty are overweight. It would be interesting to know if overweight men have less sex activity than men of optimum weight, but I have no evidence.

The most important benefit of a good sex life is the improved relationship between you and your sex partner. Although our society places a high value on romance—tenderness, consideration, and the ineffable feelings of love—it can wither rapidly in the face of poor sexual adjustment. If you want to keep romance alive, you have to keep sex alive, and—without question—vice versa. But no amount of tender feeling can by itself overcome a longstanding sexual inadequacy. You have to learn how to perform sexually for maximum benefit, just as you had to learn to eat; and you have to unlearn bad sex habits, just as you have to unlearn bad eating habits.

A good sex life also leads to a better disposition: if you are not frustrated, you will tend not to be irritable. Anger, mood swings, and even destructive acts can result from your sexual wants outrunning your sexual activity for a prolonged period.

Finally, there is pleasure. Sex is among the pleasantest of human activities, which is putting it mildly. Under the proper circumstances, that is, if you take precautions against venereal disease, pregnancy, and pain, sex is the safest of all activities undertaken for pure pleasure, safer than smoking or drinking. Most people want it, want more of it, want to appreciate it better, want it to last longer, and want to ensure that it will be part of their lives for as long as possible. Fortunately, science has begun to understand how to help them achieve all these goals.

Learning about Sex

In the investigation of sex behavior, psychiatrists—who up to now have dominated the field—have given almost all their attention to those individuals with severe sexual problems, emphasizing the bizarre rather than the usual. Dr. Kinsey, more than any other scientist in this century, changed that emphasis by studying ordinary people. The conclusion that he and his followers reached is that sexual behavior is a learned behavior, shaped by early sex experience, social standards, and biological drive.

As I have suggested, the sex act is not totally instinctive. You have to learn to do it, and you can learn it badly or you can learn it well. Even animals learn the sex act. If you raise a tomcat in isolation from other cats, he will be unable to perform the sex act with a female cat in heat. He will make some thrusting movements but will not be able to complete the mating, apparently because he missed the step-by-step learning process that takes place as cats grow up and play rough-and-tumble with each other.

Human beings also go through a step-by-step learning process, which begins early in life. They show their particular susceptibility to learning by the degree to which they develop the ability to think, talk, and dream. They also acquire attitudes, all of which are inculcated by parents, friends, and society. Sometimes the parental instruction is explicit: "Nice girls don't . . ." or "If you touch that thing, you will get a disease." There are also silent instructions: things implied but not spoken, embarrassed silences, looks of disapproval at sexual references or acts that have sexual overtones.

Children's play, also part of the overall learning process, has sexual components. Rough-and-tumble antics, flirting, curiosity about sex organs, kissing, hugging—all are activities that add to the store of sexual information. Those acts that are rewarded by approval, reciprocation, or sensual response tend to be sought after repeatedly. Those that are punished by disapproval, rejection, or lack of sensual response tend not to be repeated.

The experiences of early sex encounters can shape the adult sex pattern drastically. Suppose a teen-age male has intercourse under conditions where speed is called for—in the back of an automobile or in the young woman's home, with parents or others expected momentarily. Later on, even when there is no need to hurry, the chances are that the man will continue to have an orgasm quickly. Similar situations occur for women.

Besides being dependent on parents and friends, the complex sex-learning process is affected by the social standards at work in the community where the individual is brought up. If he is reared in an atmosphere of religious strictness, for example, where girls and boys are kept away from each other, opportunities for early sex play will be minimal; as a result there is likely to be less sex later on in life. Indeed, Kinsey and others found that adults who had been raised as believing Jews or Roman Catholics reported much less sexual activity than persons of liberal religious upbringing. Orthodox and fundamentalist groups keep adolescent boys and girls apart, emphasize the sinful aspects of nonmarital sex, and generally disapprove of sex except for the purpose of procreation. Sex for pleasure? Only if it serves to reinforce marital ties.

There is controversy about whether people are born with different sex drives. Many are easily and often aroused; others seem not to care at all and can go for months, even years, without so much as a flicker of interest. Such differences may be related to the degree of sex-hormone production, but there is no absolute proof.

As I mentioned earlier, good health improves sexual performance. If you are ill, your sex drive declines. It drops, too, as you get older, the peak for men being around the age of nineteen, for women somewhere in the twenties. This sexual fading with age may be the result of weight gain—men and women become more sedentary as they get older—of a general decline in physical condition, and, in men, of a drop in the production of certain hormones.

Although there is little chance at present of changing your basic heredity, there are some things you can improve from the biological point of view. Exercise will reduce fatigue, increase the physical ability to perform the somewhat strenuous act of love, and serve also to keep your weight down. Some physicians favor hormone therapy but its value for reviving sexuality is dubious, although the treatment has other values for older people.

Whether your sex drive is strong or weak, training can either increase or decrease your sexual performance as to frequency, intensity, nature, and duration—your sexual FIND. If your sex drive is strong, you probably cannot depress your sex activity much. If your drive is weak, there is an upper limit to how much you can improve your sex FIND, but it can be done.

What Kind of Sex Behavior Is "Right"?

The words sinful and immoral describe acts prohibited by a religion or by some sort of moral code. Clearly, what may be immoral or sinful to one person may not be so to another, whose religion or moral code is different.

Some people define the morality of a sex act according to whether it is "natural" or "unnatural." Indeed, some state laws mention unnatural acts. But what is a natural sex act? Is it an act that an individual would perform if he were not contaminated by society, like a baby feeding at the breast? Hardly. Sex research seems to have demonstrated that sex, particularly among humans, is essentially a learned behavior. Only the crudest outline of sex—touching, thrusting, ejaculation, orgasm—is instinctive. But the how of sex is learned, and thus will necessarily vary somewhat from one person to another. What is natural, then, will also vary with each individual.

Sometimes a natural sex act is defined as one that leads to procreation, because, it is argued, animals (who are "natural") perform the sex act only for procreative purposes. Actually, animals perform all sorts of sex behaviors, many of which are not directly related to making offspring. Animals perform mouth-genital contact. Males often mount males. There is anal intercourse, and not by accident, either. Human beings, even more than animals, involve themselves in sex for pleasure. Only people who deny pleasure or interpersonal communication on a sexual level would brand sex for pleasure "unnatural."

I could go on listing "definitions" of natural sex acts (there are even those who would hold that a human sex act is *un*natural when it resembles what animals do!). The point is that what you decide is natural or unnatural reflects what you have learned about sex. Your parents and peers, and society, have taught you a whole repertoire of words—"dirty," "unnatural," "abnormal," "queer"—to keep you away from acts that they have defined as illegal, immoral, or sinful.

Another way in which people show their attitude toward a particular sex behavior is to qualify it as "normal" or "abnormal." But again, the exact meaning of the term varies according to who is using it.

For scientists a behavior is normal in a statistical sense: it is average for a group. For instance, Kinsey found that forty-year-old males perform sexual intercourse with their wives about three times a week, on the average. Some men were more active, some less. Are they then abnormal? Yes, but only with reference to a particular study of behavior frequency. No moral or ethical conclusions about their behavior can or should be drawn.

"Normal" and "abnormal" are also used when characterizing biological or psychological functioning. The normal functioning of a kidney, for example, means that the kidney is excreting the right amount of water and chemicals so that body function is not impaired. There is no ideal kidney function, however; the human body can work quite well under a wide range of conditions. Abnormality is relative to the degree beyond which the body can no longer accept malfunction.

In behavior, "normal" and "abnormal" become even more tangled, because the boundary between unimpaired and impaired function depends upon what social context the individual is in and who is looking at him. Certain sex behavior on the part of a Roman Catholic girl will impair her relationship with her parents. The same behavior might be considered harmless, might even be encouraged, in a non-Roman Catholic family. It really comes down to the individual's assessment of what kind of sex behavior is likely to be socially and psychologically injurious.

Certainly we cannot be physically injured by too much sex. Males cannot perform sexual intercourse endlessly, because their ability to become aroused to erection diminishes with each successive act during a given hour or day. In females, extended sex activity may lead, temporarily, to a dry vagina, which makes intercourse difficult. Prolonged masturbation will cause an irritated penis or vagina.

The infliction of pain can produce a sexual response; indeed, for some people it is the required concomitant to sex. So there are some sexual acts that produce physical injury, and such pain or injury can impair functioning. Also, it goes beyond what most people want.

Such deviations as rape and sex acts between adults and children can produce grave psychological and physical injury. Homosexuality is another matter. The enlightened view suggests that homosexual acts between consenting adults in private carry no social dangers. However, homosexual behavior can inflict severe psychological damage in the individual if such behavior runs deeply against the beliefs of parents, friends, and community. Indeed, the problems faced by homosexuals lie not in the acts themselves, but in the participants' ability to deal with those acts psychologically and socially.

What is important to consider as part of a healthy approach to sex is this: any sex behavior is biologically and psychologically permissible, or "right," so long as it does not produce severe pain or injury—physical or psychological—in oneself or others. If you can accept this idea, you can open up possibilities for increasing your sex FIND.

Accepting New Ideas

If you decide to change your sexual pattern, your chances of success will increase dramatically if you use behavior-modification and habit-learning methods. There is a parallel with losing weight. Most people emphasize a diet—the food—but the more important aspect of a weight-loss program is learning to change your eating behavior. In the solving of sex problems, too much stress is placed on the various aspects of technique—positions, caresses, erogenous zones, performance. Not enough, if any, attention is given to learning a new behavior. As with all habit changes, particularly those of long standing, there are no miracles. It takes time, effort, and attention to detail.

Sex behavior is shaped by your attitude toward it. For example, some readers will find themselves involuntarily rejecting the contents of this chapter. They may have especially strong reactions to specific words, even though those words are in a scientific context, or they balk at taking the sex-behavior assessment. Some will be horrified at imagining oral-genital caresses, considering such acts unnatural, immoral, sinful, or illegal. At best, they may say that nice people don't do such things. Such negative attitudes can become punishments to deter behavior.

Suppose during sex play your partner asks or indicates that you touch his or her genitals with your mouth; your mental image of being arrested for the act, or of your parents' finding out, or of being punished by God, or of the penis or vagina as being in some way "dirty," can be strong enough to switch off the behavior. You will recall that a punishment works best in stopping behavior if it occurs just after the stimulus and prior to the actual behavior, and also that an aversive thought—a negative attitude—can often be a punishment.

If the sex standards of your parents, friends, and community have worked themselves into your mind in such a way as to become a series of thought punishments for various sex behaviors, or even for sex generally, your chances of carrying out those behaviors are greatly impeded. Of course, there are always those who go against the prevailing mores of the community because either they have a strong biological sex drive or they are in some way highly rewarded by the prohibited sex act. We will discuss this second reason later, when we look at the role of fantasy in sex behavior.

So, if you want to change your sex behavior, to increase your sex FIND, you may have to learn some new ideas about what may be "right" and "wrong" about sex. If you have strong religious beliefs that are in conflict with a variety of sex behaviors, you may have grave difficulty in simultaneously accepting new sex ideas, performing new sexual acts, and holding on to your religious beliefs. Keep in mind that while many people believe it is sinful to practice sexual intercourse in any position other than the face-to-face, most religions do permit variations. People tend to assume a more conservative view than their religion actually holds.

Obviously, if you want to move toward increasing the quality and quantity of sex in your life but your head is full of punishment ideas, it is not going to be easy. To help you discover just how difficult it will be for you to accept new ideas in sex, I have put together the following test. The left-hand column lists a number of sex acts performed by consenting adults in private. Circle the numbers according to how you feel about *imagining* yourself doing each act, and about others' *doing* it. All of these acts are biologically harmless if done with care; thus physical danger should not be a factor in your reactions.

Accepting Sexual Ideas

SEXUAL ACT BETWEEN CONSENTING ADULTS IN PRIVATE	*Can imagine yourself doing*			*Would object to others' doing*		
	Yes	*Maybe*	*No*	*No*	*Maybe*	*Yes*
Using sex photographs to arouse partner or self	0	1	2	0	1	2
Masturbating to orgasm	0	1	2	0	1	2
Using a mechanical vibrator to masturbate	0	1	2	0	1	2
Fondling partner's genitals	0	1	2	0	1	2
Mouth contact on partner's genitals	0	1	2	0	1	2
Penis entering vagina from the rear	0	1	2	0	1	2
Sexual acts between members of the same sex	0	1	2	0	1	2
Anal intercourse	0	1	2	0	1	2
Intercourse with animals	0	1	2	0	1	2

To score, add up the circled numbers for each column. If you score above 4 or 5 points for the last column, there is much in your upbringing that won't permit you to consider sexual ideas for others, much less yourself. You have strong ideas about what should or should not be done sexually, and will probably have trouble just considering any steps to take to increase your FIND.

If you cannot imagine yourself doing even one of the acts listed, you may have difficulty expanding your sexual horizons. Remember, this test merely asks you to imagine doing sexual acts.

Of course, you can change—if you want to. Indeed, there are programs springing up in different parts of the country designed to improve one's openness to sexual ideas. Such programs include the showing of films depicting sexual acts. (One such group of films was made by a Methodist church.) The films are shown with the intention of reducing the idea that such acts are abnormal, dirty, or strange, and of thereby opening up the viewer's acceptance of a more varied sex life.

You can change on your own by using the relaxation technique. First, relax. Next, attempt to imagine the prohibited scene. If it disturbs you, stop the thought. Imagine a less disturbing scene and then try the scene you want to imagine again. Do this until the prohibited scene is no longer disturbing. As you proceed, you will find yourself becoming sexually aroused, which is the whole idea. That scene can then be used to arouse yourself for sex.

Dealing with Failure

Failure is the biggest risk in attempting to change your sex pattern. And the worst of it is that if you fail to become aroused in a particular situation, your chances of not being aroused subsequently in the same situation are increased.

But one failure need not guarantee future failure. In attempting to relieve serious sex problems, Dr. Masters and Mrs. Johnson scrupulously guard against subjecting their patients to the possibility of failure. They use the familiar behavior-modification technique of approximating the desired behavior. Just as one does not begin an exercise program by running ten miles at full speed the first day, so one does not start a sex-improvement program by attempting a projected goal, say, of multiple orgasm on the first try. In exercise the idea is to guard against pain; in sex improvement it is to guard against potential failure. In treating a man who has difficulty in sustaining an erection, for example, Masters and Johnson do not permit in the early phases of therapy any attempt at intercourse. They prescribe instead a series of graded sexual exercises, each of which is likely to end successfully, that is, with pleasant reinforcing sensations. One small success leads to another.

Success in sex is anything that provides enjoyment, closeness, communication. Suppose you and your partner have decided to increase the number of times per week you have sexual intercourse, and on a particular night one or both of you are just too tired. Rather than push forward to meet the quota, you should fall back to hugging and kissing. Or if the situation is such that one partner does not want intercourse, he might help the other achieve a higher level of sexual release, including orgasm, accomplishing this either manually or by oral-genital contact. In short, the goal can be whatever you think will bring satisfaction—success—within a particular context. Intercourse, with or without orgasm, is only one of several goal possibilities: expressing feelings of warmth, love, amusement, relaxation in other ways can be just as satisfying on certain occasions.

What to Do about the Risk of Pregnancy

For both the unmarried and the married, fear of pregnancy can cause a series of thought punishments that inhibit sexual behavior—although Norman Mailer and others have argued the other way, that is, the element of risk of conceiving a child heightens sexual intensity. That may well be for individuals who are thrilled by risk-taking per se. But I suspect that most people would rather eliminate the risk than limit their sexual activity. This would seem to be borne out by the explosion in the use of contraceptives in this country, particularly those that remove the act of initiating contraception from the time of the sex act. From a behavioral point of view, that makes sense, because it removes aversive (fear-of-pregnancy) thoughts from the sexual response. In order of their behavioral significance, here are the contraceptives available to you:

THE PILL is a sex hormone taken by the woman for a number of days each month, depending on the type of pill, and then not taken for a few days; the cycle is repeated: so many days on, so many off. The hormone prevents ovulation (the production of an egg), which is a process essential for conception to take place. The hormone in no way interferes with sexual behavior, although some women have reported a reduction in sex drive, others an increase. The Pill may cause water retention, which makes bosoms larger and adds water weight. There is also some danger of blood clots and stroke, but the risk is low, lower than the health risks that accompany pregnancy. There are ongoing research efforts to produce less potentially damaging substances.

STERILIZATION, like the pill, is a contraceptive method that is remote in time from the sex act. By a simple surgical procedure, the sperm, in men, are prevented from leaving the penis, or the egg, in women, is prevented from reaching the womb. The surgery is essentially permanent: once you have gone through with it, you have only a 1-in-5 chance for a successful reversal procedure. Some physicians say they can reattach the tubes 40 per cent of the time; don't count on it. Thus it is not recommended for young people who intend to have children eventually. It is a safe method, and one that is becoming increasingly popular with people over forty who no longer desire to have children.

THE INTRA-UTERINE DEVICE (IUD) is a piece of plastic shaped into a coil or loop that fits into the mouth of the uterus—the cervix. Placed there by a physician, it can remain for months, even years. Like the first two, the IUD has the advantage of not interrupting the sex act. It can be removed in case pregnancy is desired. There is no hormone change. There are disadvantages: it must be inserted by a physician; the uterus can expel the IUD unbeknownst to the wearer; the IUD can—in rare instances, too rare to worry about—puncture the womb wall and produce a serious injury. Certain IUD's are not recommended for women who have never been pregnant; there are others that can be used by such women. The doctor should know which to prescribe.

THE DIAPHRAGM is a rubber or plastic disk, up to four inches in diameter, that caps the opening of the womb. It must be fitted by a physician. After applying sperm-killing cream to the diaphragm, the woman inserts it when she anticipates intercourse. Probably the most likely reason for diaphragm "failure" is that the woman fails to use it. A good way to avoid failure is to insert the diaphragm every day at the same time, whether or not there is to be sex. It can be done an hour or so before the usual most likely time for intercourse. Used in this way, it has the added advantage of separating the contraception method from the sex act. Biological problems are rare.

THE CONDOM is a rubber sheath that fits over the entire penis. It is effective, but many men complain that it interferes with sexual sensations and disturbs the mood. Since it cannot be put on until erection has been attained, it is easy to see why this is so. (It has been recorded that when the female places the condom on the penis, an extra feeling of arousal occurs.) Upon completion of intercourse the penis must be carefully withdrawn from the vagina lest the contents of the condom inadvertently spill into the vagina.

GELS, CREAMS, TABLETS, AND FOAMS, chemicals placed in the vagina just prior to intercourse to block and immobilize the sperm so that they cannot enter the womb and fertilize the egg, can be employed some time before intercourse is expected. Some couples find they produce an unpleasant sensation of slipperiness. They can be effective, but the failure rate is relatively high, compared with the other contraceptive methods so far mentioned. In combination with the condom, the chemicals are very effective.

RHYTHM is a contraceptive method based on the fact that a woman ovulates once a month and the egg is in a position to be fertilized for only three days, give or take a day. There are thus about twenty-five days in which intercourse can occur without danger of conception. It is possible to determine the time of ovulation by counting back fifteen days from the expected onset of menstruation and establishing a danger period of five days during which intercourse is eschewed. To play even safer, it has been suggested that one count back sixteen days and avoid intercourse for nine. However, because so many women have irregular menstrual cycles, the failure rate is high, to say nothing of the aversive thought that occurs concerning the ever-present risk of pregnancy.

A variation of the technique requires the woman to take her temperature with a thermometer every morning. When the temperature drops, ovulation is just about to occur or has occurred. The danger period then follows for at least eight or nine days.

WITHDRAWAL of the penis from the vagina before ejaculation theoretically prevents sperm from entering the vagina. However, many males do not have adequate control over the ejaculatory process to achieve complete withdrawal. Furthermore, there can be leakage of the sperm from the end of the penis prior to withdrawal and before ejaculation. Forget it.

You will notice that I have made only the most general statements about effectiveness of the various contraceptives. That is because measures of effectiveness are both complex and uncertain. All contraceptives have two such measures: theoretical and functional. The theoretical effectiveness is determined from studies done on animals and small groups of human beings. Functional effectiveness is derived from population studies; it depends on how many individuals in the population actually use the contraceptive and use it properly.

Dr. Christopher Tietze, one of the world's leading experts on this question, avoids figures that give a measure of the effectiveness of any contraceptive. Instead, he groups them into four clusters: most effective, highly effective, less effective, and least effective. I have summarized his conclusions, along with my estimate of behavioral effectiveness, that is, the usefulness of a particular contraceptive in promoting good sexual responses by separating initiation of contraception from the sexual act.

Effectiveness of Contraceptives

Contraceptive	Theoretical	Functional	Behavioral
Surgical sterilization	+ + + +	+ + + +	+ + + +
Oral hormones (the Pill)	+ + + +	+ + + +	+ + + +
Intra-uterine device (IUD)	+ + +	+ + + +	+ + + +

Contraceptive	Theoretical	Functional	Behavioral
Diaphragm	+++	+++	+++
Condom	+++	++	++
Foams, gels, tablets, creams	++	+++	++
Withdrawal	++	+	+
Rhythm			
Calendar	++	++	+
Temperature	++++	++	+
Postcoitus douching	+	++	++
Prolonged breast feeding of infant	+	++	+++

++++ : most effective   +++ : highly effective
++ : less effective   + : least effective

Abortion

If contraception fails and pregnancy results, then abortion becomes a real choice for many women. Following the United States Supreme Court decision of 1973, any pregnant woman is entitled to a legal abortion in the first three months of her pregnancy. It becomes more difficult to obtain one later on, but she is limited only by the consent of a physician, the facilities available, and her own sense of what an abortion might mean physically, psychologically, or morally.

In the early months of pregnancy, an abortion is safer than a tonsillectomy. It is usually performed by the aspiration method: a vacuum pump attached to a thin plastic tube extracts the contents of the uterus. Abortions become progressively less safe as the pregnancy continues, but still it remains one of the safest medical procedures.

It is not good sense—in my view—to rely on abortion, permitting oneself to become lax in the application of a contraceptive. First, it can be expensive, up to seven hundred dollars—although in New York City it has been possible to obtain abortions for as little as one hundred and thirty-five dollars. I suspect the price will come down as other physicians around the country take up the practice. I see no reason why, in 1973, an abortion in the first three months of pregnancy should not cost fifty dollars.

Second, despite all the rationalizations about the impersonal nature of an abortion, it is still for most women a chilling experience. In some clinics, special counseling can be obtained to lessen the impact; but many physicians refuse to lighten the load on the woman and indeed often generate feelings of guilt, panic, and fear in her.

Third, these circumstances or even the thought of such possibilities can depress a woman's sex desires. I should add that it is probable that a man faced with the fact that his sex partner needs an abortion also experiences a cooling of ardor; estrangement can result.

One can only conclude that while abortion in the 1970's removes much of the fear of having out-of-wedlock or unwanted children, a fear that was rampant in the days of illegal abortions, contraception offers a safer and more sensible route of avoiding pregnancy.

Venereal Disease

The late 1960's and the early 1970's saw a dramatic rise in the number of cases of syphilis and gonorrhea in the United States. Public-health officers declared gonorrhea out of control, with estimates that one woman out of every ten who was having regular intercourse was infected. The general rise in sexual activity, particularly as characterized by one individual's having a variety of sex partners, is one reason for the increase in VD cases. Another is that fewer men use the condom, which protects against both syphilis and gonorrhea. It has been suggested that the Pill makes the tissues of the vagina more susceptible to infection. Also to be considered is the fact that jet air travel has become a commonplace in our lives. Thus, large numbers of people are constantly moving from one part of the country to another; inevitably some carry VD with them. Outbreaks of VD can spring up anywhere, any time.

The problem of VD is real enough; but fear has been used to prevent sexual activity. Indeed, the entire VD-education program, because it is aimed at controlling venereal disease, stresses the importance of stopping sexual activity and getting to a doctor for treatment. Such a nonconstructive program must eventually fail—as, I think, this one has. A particularly unfortunate result is that now many people's sexual behavior is burdened with yet another aversive thought: sex is connected with disease.

There are ways to prevent venereal disease in the first place. One is to have intercourse with one partner and one only. The more partners you have the more risk you run. Another preventive measure is washing. If both partners wash their genitals before and after intercourse, they will reduce the germ population and, with that, the possibility of infection, should one partner have a venereal disease. To avoid a possible feeling of insult in case only one partner washes, the partners can wash each other. This provides not only protection, but also a sense of closeness and sexual fun. Urination immediately after intercourse has a cleansing effect in that it rinses germs out of the tube leading to the bladder.

Chemicals have been developed that, when deposited in the vagina, will kill venereal disease germs. While successful in preliminary trials, such chemicals are not yet available on the open market. However, since contraceptive creams apparently have some germ-killing power, a woman could at least partially protect herself against VD by using one of the creams, gels, tablets, or foams.

Homosexuals should be particularly aware of the preventive measure of washing; it has been shown that their sexual lives are more likely to be characterized by venereal infection than are those of heterosexuals. This is probably related to the fact that homosexuals generally have a much greater variety of sex partners than do heterosexuals.

Extramarital and Nonmarital Intercourse

Twenty years ago, Dr. Kinsey reported that at least half the married men and a quarter of the women had sex relations with persons other than their spouses at least once in their lifetimes. There are some experts who believe that the figures are higher today, although not dramatically so.

We are in the midst of constantly increasing and widening sexual activity. I believe that one of the major factors contributing to this increased activity is the new mobility of women. In the past, women were more or less isolated from men in the community, except, of course, at those public gatherings that were socially sanctioned, such as church. Today almost half of the married women in the United States are in the labor force; daily meetings with men outside of their immediate circle of friends and family are common. In such circumstances—especially in large cities, where meetings are frequent and simple—one would expect a rise in extramarital intercourse.

Although most religious codes uniformly condemn it, extramarital intercourse continues on an ever-increasing scale. Though we may be reluctant to admit it, extramarital sexual activity may have reached the stage where it has the appeal of a fashion: "Everybody's doing it . . . why not me?" If that is the case, we can expect an explosion of extramarital sex within two decades, unless some social pressure intervenes.

Under present social conditions, many individuals who attempt extramarital intercourse find themselves in one or more of the following difficulties:

• They experience feelings of psychological guilt, often in combination with religious remorse, which can impair social functioning. Most of the time the guilt or remorse is temporary; much depends on the way in which the individual was reared. For some people the psychological consequences are permanent.

• They become deeply involved with the extramarital partner and get into marital difficulty—a factor in the ever-rising divorce rate.

• They contract a venereal disease.

• The affair results in pregnancy. This is not as much of a problem as it once was, with legal abortions becoming more widely available and knowledge of effective contraception being almost universal.

• Extramarital relations become a habit; interest in solving any marital sex problems declines.

• Extramarital relations are used as a weapon in a psychological war against one's marriage partner.

These difficulties are not trivial. Any one of them could be catastrophic, psychologically, socially, economically. Few know in advance if they are going to be able to manage an extramarital relationship successfully.

Sooner or later the possibility of extramarital sexual relations will probably present itself to you, as it has to an ever-increasing number of people; it is a good idea to consider beforehand what the disadvantages and advantages might be. Instead of allowing circumstances alone to govern your decision, try to approach the situation rationally. I have already pointed out some of the difficulties; here are some positive aspects to consider:

• An extramarital sexual relationship can provide a sexual outlet for someone whose spouse has a low sex interest or capacity.

• It can provide new interest in sexual activity for many individuals who find that their marital sex activity is on the wane.

• It can be an opportunity to acquire new sexual or interpersonal skills, which might be applied to one's own marriage.

• Establishing intimacy with more than one person can broaden one's psychological horizons.

• Extramarital intercourse can mean a renewed spirit of sexual adventure and a reawakened interest in one's physical condition.

• It can provide the psychic motivation to refurbish a failing marriage by forcing one to examine the marriage for its strengths as well as its weaknesses.

If you do opt for extramarital activity, remember to be very cautious about any decision to tell your spouse. Regardless of how sophisticated you think your marital partner may be, regardless of the number of times you have discussed the problem in the abstract and have said that it wouldn't matter, most experts agree that in almost all cases it *does* matter. Most Americans cannot withstand the reality of extramarital sex by their spouses—and men are the more vulnerable to such disclosures.

Should single men and women engage in sex? The question sounds old-fashioned today, although most religious and social codes say no, particularly for women. Sex is especially disapproved of when done for profit or exploitation, when one partner is much younger than the other, or when the partners are of the same sex. Your attitude will depend on your upbringing.

Occasionally one still hears the argument that for the young, particularly women, premarital intercourse interferes with marriage. But the evidence suggests that premarital sex causes trouble only if the male has a strict code of virginity for his bride or if he believes strongly that it is "not nice" for his wife to have slept around.

Kinsey suggested, and there is no recent evidence to the

contrary, that women who have had orgasm before marriage, and particularly orgasm in intercourse, are more likely to have orgasm in marriage and to be more sexually attuned in general. On the other hand, if a woman "saves" herself for her husband, she does not really seem to be saving very much, unless she places a great value on monogamy and has prepared herself for the sexual part of marriage. If this is not true, she risks delivering herself as a sexually inadequate, fearful, and repressed wife.

Nonmarital sex is not without risks—pregnancy, venereal disease, failure. The last, of course, can damage the future sex behavior of an individual. Someone who engages in many sexual adventures while young, without learning how to develop an intimate relationship, has learned sexual technique but has missed the psychological pleasures of close communication.

Sex-Monitoring

Suppose that now you wish to change your sex frequency, intensity, nature, or duration. Let's start with frequency: you have decided that you want to increase the number of times a week you have intercourse with your partner. The first step is for both of you to decide your goal together; otherwise there is a danger that the nonparticipating partner will be resentful, causing the whole procedure to backfire.

One of the most useful behavior-modification techniques is self-monitoring, as you will have seen from reading the chapters on exercise and work habits. Self-monitoring means that you keep a written record of what you are doing. Dr. Jay Mann and his associates at the University of California Medical Center, San Francisco, showed pornographic movies to sexually normal couples. The couples were also asked to write down and keep track of all sexual activities. The act of self-monitoring was more effective in increasing sex activity than the pornographic movies.

As you and your partner begin your self-monitoring, remember that it is important to go slowly. Failure is a great deterrent to sex. If you and your partner seek a high level of performance almost immediately, you are bound to fail if you try to quickly close a large gap between what you are doing and what you want to achieve. You must approach your distant goal slowly, by approximation, just as you would with exercise, dieting, and work habits. You will be trying to learn a new habit pattern in one of the most delicately balanced of all human activities.

Or suppose you and your partner are having sexual intercourse once a week and your sex-behavior assessment indicates that you both want to have intercourse three times a week. The first thing to consider is the conditions under which you now have intercourse. Is it a time when both of you are rested—say, on Sundays when neither of you works? Then you should reduce your fatigue during the week. There can be several reasons for undue fatigue: consistently working late, lack of daily exercise, overweight— sometimes the fatigue people feel in the late evening is nothing more than the result of a long, heavy dinner. Or you can go to bed one or two hours earlier on the days you want to have intercourse.

Try making a date with your spouse to have sex, just as you would make a date to go out to dinner. Make the date early in the same day or even the day before. That gives you both a chance to think about sex, which can help create a mood that is conducive to sexual activity.

Your first approximation to increased sexual behavior can be merely to get into bed and have some prolonged sex play. You can massage each other, talk intimately, discuss the kinds of things you like to do sexually. You should enjoy the session, even if intercourse does not occur.

If you have more than two or three such sex dates during the week without trying to have intercourse, you will find that on one or more of those occasions you will end by having it or one or both of you may experience orgasm without intercourse— through manual manipulation or oral contact.

All the while you should keep track of what has been happening to you sexually. One easy way is to keep a sex diary: monitoring each day's sexual events will work for you and your partner.

Another easy way to keep track is to use a chart like the one shown. The *x*'s represent sex dates with your partner, the *o*'s are days of sexual intercourse, and the boxed letters on Saturdays represent the total for the week. Connecting the boxed letters with a line will give you a quick visual record of your progress. The chart is nothing more or less than a reminder and, like other self-

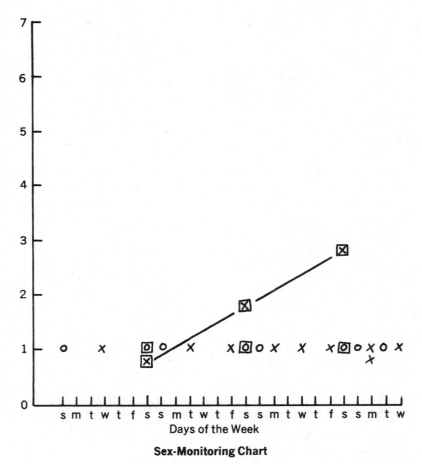

Sex-Monitoring Chart

monitoring devices, it provides a generalized reward for habitual-izing a new behavior.

Sexual Outlet

In American society sexual intercourse with orgasm seems to have been placed above all other kinds of sexual contact or activity. For most people it is the only desired end. However, there is also a spectrum of sexual activity that includes masturbation, heavy petting to orgasm, necking without orgasm, homosexual acts, oral-genital sex, et cetera. Dr. Kinsey and his colleagues recorded the number of times the people they interviewed engaged in any kind of sexual activity and the sum of those activities was called "sexual outlet." They found men who seemed quite content with masturbating three times a day, engaging in no other sex activity; there were others who enjoyed mostly oral sex. The range was tremendous.

Not all the sex acts listed above may be to your liking, but for many people they are pleasurable. As I have said, it all depends on what you have learned to like (as with food) and on what type of partner is available to you. Masturbation—self-stimulation—has much to recommend it. It is convenient; it can be fast or slow; it does not require a partner. It is safe from the point of view of venereal disease and pregnancy. Masturbation is the only or most enjoyable way that many women can achieve orgasm. And, as Dr. Masters and Mrs. Johnson have shown, the physical response to masturbation is more intense than it is to sexual intercourse. Masturbation provides for good sex practice. Its chief drawback is, of course, that it precludes the satisfaction of an intimate interpersonal relationship.

Restricting your sexual activity to intercourse may deprive you, first, of a variety of pleasure and, second, of enough sexual activity to keep your interest in sex at a sufficiently high level for your needs. Contrary to popular myth, holding back on sex does not necessarily increase desire—just the opposite may be true in the long run. An increase in one sex activity may lead to an increase in other sex activities. One reason for this is that by doing different things, the signals, or stimuli, for sex become more varied. And fantasy plays a role in starting and continuing sexual behavior.

The Power of Fantasy

Most people have daydreams—fantasies—during sexual activity. While having intercourse with his wife, a man may conjure up a vision of another woman, without any the less loving his wife. Or when he is in one position, he may imagine himself in another. A woman may have an impression of being in another place—near the ocean or in the country. Fantasies are most common during masturbation. There is a growing feeling among sex therapists that the ability to fantasize improves one's capacity to be aroused and to achieve satisfactory sexual responses.

It may be worthwhile to practice sex fantasy for this purpose. There is nothing wrong with purposely enjoying sex thoughts. But if you find that they are punishing thoughts, try offsetting this effect by using the relaxation technique. When you are completely relaxed, allow yourself to imagine a sexual scene. If it disturbs you, stop the thought and try another, one less troubling. Approximate the sexual-thought goal in this way, step by step. Whatever thought arouses you sexually without troubling you is an effective sex fantasy.

If you have sex fantasies during intercourse, let them ride if they help you to keep the sex act going. A warning: do not share them with your partner, lest they be interpreted as a criticism. For example, if you happen to imagine another person during intercourse and you tell your partner about it, your partner may think or even say: "What's the matter? Am I not sexy enough?" Such a reaction is likely to be far from your intention in revealing your fantasy.

The power of fantasy can under certain circumstances be quite impressive, as recent research suggests. The experiment involved men who engaged in homosexual or fetishistic (in which the erotic interest is focused on a part of the body or an article of clothing) activity while actually wanting to have heterosexual activity; yet they could not be aroused by women. The treatment depended on the most powerful reward in sex: orgasm. If orgasm occurs, the behavior that immediately precedes it is likely to recur in the future, a conclusion that is no surprise to readers of this book. Here is how the researchers used this fact.

Each patient was instructed to masturbate as he usually did, that is, employing homosexual or fetishistic fantasies to arouse himself. Then, just at the moment of orgasm, he was asked to switch his fantasy to a scene of himself with a woman in sexual contact and to keep that picture alive in his mind during orgasm. Each man did the act in private.

Once a patient was able to picture a woman when he was at the point of orgasm, he was told to bring up the scene a little earlier—say twenty seconds. If he could then picture the woman and still be aroused up to and including orgasm, he was told to imagine the heterosexual scene forty seconds earlier. In this way the patient worked his way back in time with his heterosexual fantasy. At each stage the scene aroused him because it was ultimately followed by the rewarding orgasm. Eventually, every man in the group could arouse himself and masturbate to orgasm with heterosexual fantasy. After that was achieved, each of them tried to engage in heterosexual intercourse (again in a stepwise fashion, using the behavior-modification technique of approximation). With this method, twelve out of the fourteen men who wanted to have heterosexual relationships learned to do so.

Following the lesson of that experiment, you can learn to arouse yourself using sexual ideas previously unappealing to you. Perhaps your goal is oral-genital sex play; daydreaming about it can help you overcome any resistance you have to trying it. Eventually, daydreams, if they are arousing, thus act as thought rewards. But sometimes you do not want your dream act to occur. For example, you may not want to really engage in extramarital sex. My interviews with sex therapists indicate that if an act is beyond the realm of real possibility for an individual, fantasy alone will not lead him into it. For instance, many men who have homosexual fantasies are frightened; they feel that it must mean that they either are homosexual or really want to have homosexual activities. Neither is necessarily true; if homosexual activity is beyond your real needs, there is little chance of your actually engaging in it.

Now, suppose that you are a married man and your problem is that you have difficulty being sexually aroused by your wife. If you are already having intercourse with her without difficulty, make a concerted effort at the point of orgasm, in intercourse or masturbation, to imagine your wife's face or body or genitals, even though earlier during the sex act you used other fantasies. Or you can daydream a sexual scene involving your wife at the moment of your orgasm. If you succeed in doing that, try to bring up the image of your wife a little earlier next time. If you lose erection, go back to your other daydreams and think of your wife at the moment of orgasm. By thinking of her earlier and earlier, you will eventually find that you are more and more aroused by both the thought and sight of your wife.

If you have difficulty switching your fantasies during inter-course, try doing it while masturbating or performing any other sex act that ends with an orgasm. There are many women who do not achieve orgasm in intercourse or by masturbation; but almost all women feel a sense of arousal and they can sense a peaking of that sensation. They can use that peaking sensation as a reward for a sexual fantasy. However, many inorgasmic women have achieved orgasm with mechanical vibrators, a device that could open the way to a broader sex life.

From this description of what fantasy can do, you can see that it should be used carefully. I have no evidence for it, but I suspect that if you do not want to engage in homosexual acts, it is a good idea not to fantasize them at the point of orgasm. Similarly, fantasies of physical punishment, which are arousing for many people, should not be carried forward to orgasm or peak physical arousal. In fact, all sex fantasies can be useful imaginings for the purpose of achieving arousal or freedom in sex; but be wary of approaching orgasm or peak sexual arousal with those whose activities you wish to avoid. Although fantasy can powerfully move many people to sexual arousal, it is weak for others. If this is true for you, you may find other means of increasing your sex drive—by reading, perhaps, or viewing sexually stimulating material.

Sensuality and Intensity

The lessons of behavior modification can be used to increase the intensity of your sexual life as well as the frequency. But first, it must be pointed out that how you respond to being touched is a pretty reliable indication of how you respond physically and emotionally to sex. If you tend to be unresponsive to the touch of another person's hand on you, you probably do not respond with a full range of feeling to sex. Thus if your goal is to increase the degree of intensity of your sexual activities, you may have to start out by increasing your repertoire of response to touch. Even if you wish merely to heighten your pleasure in sexual responses, such touch training can help you.

Treatment of severe sex disorders by Dr. Masters and Mrs. Johnson depends in great part on sensuality training. You can take advantage of what they have learned, applying it to your particular situation. Co-operation of your partner will make it an ideal learning experience.

You can start out by learning to stroke your partner's body in ways that give him or her pleasure. I use the word learning advisedly, because, for some peculiar reason, many people believe that their sex partners should know "instinctively" how to do this, not realizing that pleasure varies tremendously from person to person. Ask your partner to let you know what is particularly pleasing. It doesn't have to be in words; there are other means of communicating feelings—gestures, small moans, et cetera—if you think that words might interfere with the mood.

There are areas of the body—the so-called erogenous zones— that seem to respond to touch more often than others: the backs of the calves and upper arms, the inner thighs, the region between the ribs and the navel, the side of the neck. However, it is not a hard and fast rule that everybody is responsive in all these places. Thus it is my opinion that the way of finding what is best for you and your partner is to experiment, making up your own "rules" from your particular intimate experiences.

The primary goal of this exercise is for each partner to learn how to give pleasure so that he can get pleasure: Masters and Johnson call this "give to get." You should not—at first—deliberately end the stroking session with intercourse; you should just learn to appreciate the sense of touching and being touched. Set aside time for stroking, kissing, cuddling, and talk. Of course, if the session does end with intercourse or some other orgasmic act, no great harm; indeed, more power to you.

It is possible to heighten sensuality by using massage cream, available in most drugstores and at notions counters. (Steer clear of medicated creams, which often have strong odors.) Masters and Johnson have prescribed massage creams as a useful way of developing touch awareness. They have also shown that people who resist using such creams are also resistant to solving their sex problems. There are many massage books available, which could be of some help, but the best guide is your partner.

As you have probably realized by now, sensuality training

provides good practice in the kind of communication that should occur during the sex act. Many partners do not tell each other what they like or do not like. Somehow they are supposed to just know; the act of telling what feels good seems too mechanical. But remember, a failure of communication can result in sex failure.

What if you have no sex partner? You can train yourself to stroke your own body and to feel pleasure in doing so. If you accompany it with sexual fantasy, you may find yourself sexually aroused enough to masturbate.

While *The Sensuous Woman*, by J., may not be stylistically to everyone's taste, it does contain many valuable hints on self-stimulation that could be used, for example, by a woman who has difficulty achieving orgasm in intercourse. She can practice having orgasm while masturbating. If she has never had an orgasm, with or without intercourse, this again might be the answer.

Of course, the problem of the inorgasmic woman is a larger one than can be dealt with here, but masturbation is worth a try before seeking special help. The woman can also use self-monitoring and sensuality training with masturbation in her trial program for achieving orgasm. Electric vibrators and massage creams can increase the probability of orgasm's occurring.

There is also an exercise that can help to raise orgasmic probability. It was discovered quite by accident by Dr. A. H. Kegel, a California urologist. A woman patient of his could not retain urine, which he found to be caused by a weakness in the muscle controlling the flow of urine from the bladder. His prescription was an exercise designed to strengthen that muscle. The exercise not only solved her immediate problem; it also made it possible for her to achieve orgasm in intercourse, something she had never experienced. Dr. Kegel subsequently prescribed the exercise for inorgasmic women and the result was the same for many of them. The exercise strengthens the muscles of the vagina, which contributes to orgasmic potential by improving sensual response. The woman can also provide extra stimulation for her partner by contracting the vaginal muscle around the shaft of the penis.

The exercise is easy, and there are two ways to approach it: while standing, adjust the muscles in your pelvis as if you are going to urinate and then squeeze down hard as if you are trying to stop the flow; or, squeeze your anus shut as if you were trying to stop defecation. Either way, the result is contraction of the vaginal muscles.

Interestingly enough, Dr. Kegel's exercise also works for men. With practice, a man can achieve muscular control over the movement of his penis and thus be able to sustain a flagging erection. During the early phases of intercourse and after intercourse is completed, such control can give the female partner additional sensations of pleasure.

Mood

Improvement in communication will automatically heighten the mood during sexual activities. If the partners tell each other what they like before, during, and after sex, the mood can change from one characterized by urgency, speed, and physicality to one characterized by passion and a sense of deep interpersonal involvement.

Communication goes beyond sex. Time can be spent just talking about everyday things, ideas, hopes, the future. Some care has to be taken to avoid topics that might lead to arguments. It is not a good idea to get into a fight in the place where you have sex, because the room can then become a signal for argument.

Telling your partner how much you admire him or her sexually, how much you enjoy his or her company, how much you look forward to each encounter can be particularly effective before sexual contact, and also immediately following the act. Remember, praise following an act is a reward for that act and is likely to make it occur again.

Human beings take pleasure in dealing with ideas, words, and emotions. If you leave them out of your sex life, you are cheating yourself of a great deal of pleasure.

Duration

You may want to extend the duration of the sex act for many reasons: you like the sensations generated by the activity prior to orgasm and want to prolong them; you may be capable of multiple orgasms during intercourse (this is true almost exclusively of women) and want to experience them, especially if your partner takes a long time to become sexually aroused and to achieve orgasm.

Usually, the duration of intercourse centers around the man's ability to maintain an erection. That in turn depends not only on his sex drive, but on what his partner is doing. If she is quiet and reticent, his interest and erection will flag. If she is passionate, he may have an orgasm quickly. If he ejaculates and has an orgasm, there will then be a period, the refractory period, during which he will not be able to have an erection. Depending on age and circumstance, that period may last minutes, hours, or even days. The older the man, the longer the refractory period. However, the time between erections may be shortened by novel stimulation. Many men who have extramarital sexual activities discover that with the new sex partner they have orgasm more frequently and their refractory period shortens considerably. However, when the novelty of the "new woman" wears off and is not replaced by other novel stimuli, the refractory period returns to what it had been before.

Many of the suggestions in the sections about sensuality, mood, and communication can provide a variety of ever-changing stimuli, which, if properly used, can have many benefits, including the shortening of the refractory period with a longtime sex partner. With practice, a man can, for instance, lengthen the period before ejaculation by retarding orgasm. He can do this in several ways. One ancient method is to stop thinking sexual thoughts. Or he can concentrate on his sexual sensations, learning where the peaks occur and pausing to allow them to pass. Women can do the same thing to step up their sense of awareness. Another way requires mutual co-operation. Some years ago, a treatment was developed for males suffering from premature ejaculation, that is, ejaculating before the penis has entered the vagina or almost immediately thereafter. It was worked out by Dr. James Semans and later elaborated by Masters and Johnson. It depends on the observation that if at the moment just prior to ejaculation the head of the penis is squeezed, there will be no orgasm and erection will subside.

In the procedure the woman first arouses the man sexually by stroking his body or penis, or both, until he is at the point of orgasm. At that moment the man signals her and she places her thumb on the underside of his penis near the head and circles the head with her index and middle finger. She squeezes hard for three seconds. When the penis softens, the squeeze is working. If the process is repeated several times over many days, the man learns to withhold orgasm and ejaculation until he can place his penis into the vagina without rapidly ejaculating. The technique is more complicated than I have described it and requires guidance from a professional. This technique can be used to extend the duration of sexual contact. It requires some co-ordination and a mutual feeling of doing something to increase your joint pleasure and sense of control.

You can also use the method of stop-start: coming close to the peak of arousal, pausing, then starting again. You do this either by the squeeze or by concentrating on the rising feelings of arousal. Stop-start intensifies the sexual response more than any fancy ideas of position or erogenous zones.

Orgasm Is Not All

There was a time when sex manuals listed simultaneous orgasm as the primary goal in intercourse. For most people, this target is difficult to achieve, because of the variability of sexual responsiveness. Concentration on timing often has the effect of cooling sexual arousal. It is better for the couple to strive for a long-duration intercourse, because that raises the probability that both will have orgasm. One way to extend duration is to increase the amount of stroking, cuddling, kissing, and talk before attempting intercourse; another is to use stop-start.

Sometimes one partner is not interested in intercourse when the other partner is. For too many couples that spells the end of sexual contact for the day. However, if you discuss the situation beforehand, it will be possible for the partner who does not want intercourse to help the other have orgasm by some other means; each couple must discover what particularly satisfies them. For some it might be oral-genital contact; for others, stroking the genital organs. Or one partner can masturbate—stroking his or her own genitals—while the other fondles and kisses. It must be stressed that an orgasm, complete with fireworks, is simply not a necessary event every time you engage in sexual activity. Many men and women find satisfaction in a sustained period of sexual arousal. This is particularly true of people as they get older. As men age they may thrust for longer times during intercourse and not have ejaculation. This can often be quite satisfying for them, unless, of course, they are under the misapprehension that ejaculation must occur or intercourse isn't worth having—in which case they experience a profound sense of failure; this in turn makes it difficult for them to have an erection on subsequent occasions.

Even young men and women need not expect orgasm, and can, unless they are performance oriented, simply enjoy the special pleasures that the process of sexual arousal can bring.

Positions

I do not want to add to the voluminous material written about positions in intercourse. Sex manuals are available, and almost all of them are encyclopedic on the subject. If you think a particular position might be arousing and satisfying, don't hesitate to communicate that to your partner. You won't know until you try which position or positions in intercourse will be most satisfying. Position in intercourse is, in my view, the least important aspect. More attention should be given to attitude, practice, sensuality, and mood.

Summary

If you want a better sex life that lasts for a long period of your life, you can do much to achieve that goal by using the techniques of behavior modification. Physical vigor achieved by exercise and weight control can make you physically capable of carrying out the sex act more frequently, making it last longer, and also making it possible for you to have sex well into old age.

Behavior-change methods useful in sex include:

APPROXIMATION. Planning small-step improvements in frequency, intensity, and duration, rather than jumping rapidly ahead.

MONITORING. Keeping track of what you do sexually day by day and setting near-term goals.

SENSUAL TRAINING. With stroking, cuddling, and massage, you can broaden your sensitivity to touch and intensify your sexual response. Masturbation can help women who are of low orgasmic experience achieve more orgasms more easily.

FANTASY. Daydreaming can be sexually arousing—and sexual arousal can make images more exciting.

COMMUNICATION. Telling your partner what you like and vice versa can improve the sex mood as well as intensify all of the sexual sensations. Talking about ideas and things before and after intercourse can refine the interpersonal relationship.

SEXUAL TECHNIQUES. Trying various methods of stimulation can only improve your and your partner's pleasure in sexual arousal. Stop-start is an important method of increasing sensitivity.

One Last Word of Caution

Sex is one of the most delicately balanced of behaviors. It is extremely perishable under the heat of failure. As you begin your effort to improve, concentrate on using approximation, so that failures, if any, are small and not devastating.

Sexual responsiveness tends to wither if the individuals attempt mentally to observe themselves during the sex activity. Thus, when you try something new, start it and forget it; focus on the sexuality rather than on how well you are doing. For example, if you are monitoring your sexual activity by recording your sex acts in a diary or on a chart, do the recording long after the act so that you are not thinking of yourself as a performer. The monitoring acts to initiate sex, but once you start think only of your partner, your fantasies, your pleasure. Enjoy.